CBS Confident Pharmacy Series

Drug Store and Business Management

Third Edition

for Second Year Diploma in Pharmacy

(0815) Strictly Based on Syllabus as per ER1991

V.N. Raje M Pharm

Principal
Gourishankar Education Society's
GES College of Pharmacy (D Pharm)
Limb, Satara, Maharashtra

W0235508

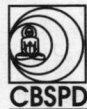

CBSPD

CBS Publishers & Distributors Pvt Ltd

New Delhi • Bengaluru • Chennai • Kochi • Kolkata • Lucknow • Mumbai
Hyderabad • Jharkhand • Nagpur • Patna • Pune • Uttarakhand

CBS Confident Pharmacy Series

Drug Store and Business Management

Third Edition

for Second Year Diploma in Pharmacy

(0815) Strictly Based on Syllabus as per ER1991

Question–Answer Type Notes and Board Question Papers (1996 to 2017)

Salient Features

- ❏ Total Confidence and 100 percent Success in Every Examination.
- ❏ Repeatedly Asked Board Questions Indicated in Brackets.
- ❏ Chapterwise Collection of Very Important Questions.
- ❏ Written in Very Simple and Lucid Language.
- ❏ Board Question Papers 2015–2017 given at the End of Text.

Drug Store and Business Management
Third Edition

ISBN: 978-93-86478-47-4

Copyright © Author and Publisher

Third Edition: 2018
  Reprint: 2018, 2019, 2020, 2021, 2022, 2024
First Edition: 2010
  Reprint: 2011
Second Edition: 2015
  Reprint: 2016

Published by Satish Kumar Jain and produced by Varun Jain for

CBS Publishers & Distributors Pvt Ltd
4819/XI Prahlad Street, 24 Ansari Road, Daryaganj, New Delhi 110 002, India
Ph: 011-23289259, 23266861   Website: www.cbspd.com
                                    e-mail: delhi@cbspd.com
Corporate Office: 204 FIE, Industrial Area, Patparganj, Delhi 110 092
Ph: 011-4934 4934   Fax: 011-4934 4935   e-mail: publishing@cbspd.com; publicity@cbspd.com

Branches

- **Bengaluru:** Seema House 2975, 17th Cross, K.R. Road, Banasankari 2nd Stage, Bengaluru 560 070, Karnataka, India
  Ph: +91-80-26771678/79   Fax: +91-80-26771680   e-mail: bangalore@cbspd.com
- **Chennai:** 7, Subbaraya Street, Shenoy Nagar, Chennai 600 030, Tamil Nadu, India
  Ph: +91-44-26680620, 26681266   Fax: +91-44-42032115   e-mail: chennai@cbspd.com
- **Kochi:** 42/1325, 1326, Power House Road, Opp KSEB, Power House, Ernakulam 682 018, Kerala, India
  Ph: +91-484-4059061-65   Fax: +91-484-4059065   e-mail: kochi@cbspd.com
- **Kolkata:** 147, Hind Ceramics Compound, 1st Floor, Nilgunj Road, Belghoria, Kolkata-700056 West Bengal, India
  Ph: 033-25633055, 033-25633056   e-mail: kolkata@cbspd.com
- **Lucknow:** Basement, Khushnuma Complex, 7-Meerabai Marg (Behind Jawahar Bhawan) Lucknow 226001, India
  Ph: 0522-4000032   e-mail: tiwari.lucknow@cbspd.com
- **Mumbai:** PWD Shed. Gala no. 25/26, Ramchandra Bhatt Marg, Next to JJ Hospital Gate no. 2, Opp. Union Bank of India Noorbaug Mumbai-400009, Maharashtra, India
  Ph: 022-66661880/89   e-mail: mumbai@cbspd.com

Representatives
- **Hyderabad** 0-9885175004 • **Jharkhand** 0-9811541605 • **Nagpur** 0-9421945513
- **Patna** 0-9334159340 • **Pune** 0-9923910676 • **Uttarakhand** 0-9716462459

Printed at Mudrak, Noida, UP, India

to
my beloved family

Preface to the Third Edition

The third edition of the now popular and successful book includes Board Question Papers 1996 to 2017. The book has been written to meet the requirements of students of Diploma in Pharmacy (D Pharm) in accordance with the new revised syllabus ER1991 prescribed by Pharmacy Council of India.

This book is small and humble effort has been put in for compiling necessary information on the subject. An attempt has been made to demystify and simplify the basic concepts for the students of pharmacy and to enable them get an evergreen success in MSBTE examinations.

The salient features of the present book are:

- Lucid and easy language,
- To the point answers,
- Remembering facts in the simplest way, and
- Infusing confidence in the reader to appear in the Board Examinations.

Hence the series is named

CBS Confident Pharmacy Series

I am confident that this book will be useful to both the students and the teachers of Diploma in Pharmacy as well as the candidates desiring to succeed in competitive examinations for better job opportunities in pharmacy profession such as hospital pharmacists in PHCs, civil hospitals, etc.

Raje Vijay N

Acknowledgements

I express my heartfelt thanks to Prof Madan Jagtap, Chairman, Gourishankar Education Society, Satara Maharashtra, for consistent encouragement and inspiration for writing this book.

I wish to acknowledge the prompt and efficient help given by Prof Milind Jagtap, Mr Jaywant Salunkhe, Mr Appa Rajage, Mr Nitin Mudalgikar, and Mr Shrirang Katekar of Gourishankar Education Society, Satara.

I am also thankful to Shri Satish Kumar Jain, Chairman and Managing Director, and Shri RN Mandal, General Manager, Pune Branch, CBS Publishers & Distributors Pvt Ltd, for their sustained efforts and keen interest in the publication of this book.

I wish all my beloved students to have a great success in the Board Examinations.

Raje Vijay N

Syllabus

(As per ER 1991)

Drug Store and Business Management

Part I: Commerce

1. Introduction: Trade, industry and commerce, functions and subdivision of commerce, introduction to elements of economics and management.
2. Forms of Business Organisation
3. Channels of Distribution
4. Drug House Management—Selection of site, space layout and legal requirements.

   Importance and objectives of purchasing, selection of suppliers, credit information, tenders, contracts and price determination and legal requirements thereto.
5. Inventory Control—Objects and importance, modern techniques like ABC, VED analysis, the lead time, inventory carrying cost, safety stock, minimum and maximum stock levels, economic order quantity, scrap and surplus disposal.
6. Sales promotion, market research, salesmanship, qualities of a salesman, advertising and window display.
7. Recruitment, training, evaluation and compensation of the pharmacist.
8. Banking and Finance Service and functions of bank. Finance planning and sources of finance.

Part II: Accountancy

1. Introduction to the accounting concepts and conventions, Double entry book keeping, Different kinds of accounts.
2. Cash book.
3. General ledger and Trial balance.
4. Profit and loss account and balance sheet.
5. Simple technique of analysing financial statements.
6. Introduction to Budgeting.

Contents

Contents

Introduction to Economics and Management

1 Define the terms.

☞ **i. Economics**

"Economics is a branch of knowledge which deals with consumption, production, exchange and distribution of wealth."

ii. Business (S. 96, 00, 03, 04, 07; W. 01, 04)

Business means any activity which involves production and distribution of goods and services with the main purpose of earning profit."

iii. Industry (S. 06; W. 03, 04, 05)

"Industry is a part of business activity which is related to activities like production, repacking, extraction, fabrication, manufacturing, processing, etc."

iv. Commerce (S. 97, 98, 00, 02, 05, 09; W. 96, 97, 98, 01, 03)

"Commerce is defined as the sum total of all activities which are engaged in removal of hindrances of person, place, time, money and others in the exchange of commodities."

"Commerce is a part of business which includes all those activities which facilitate the smooth exchange of goods and services."

v. Trade (S. 96, 97, 98, 00, 01, 02, 06; W. 97, 99, 01, 04, 05)

"The trade means buying, selling and exchange of goods and services."

vi. Aids to Trade

"The factors which remove hindrances in trading are known as aids to trade."

2 **Give the classification of various business activities. (S. 08, W. 96, 98, 99)**

☞

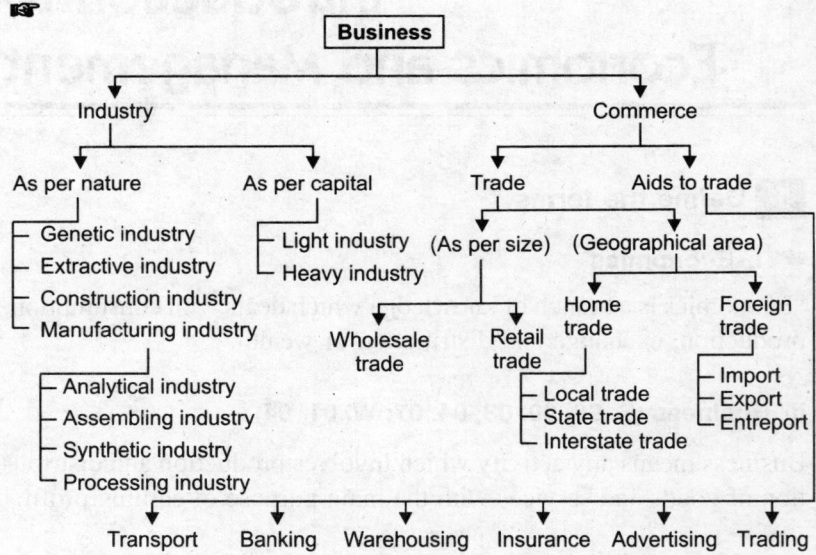

3 **Write a note on 'elements of economics'. (S. 96, 98, 00, 01, 04, 05, 09; W. 96, 00, 01)**

☞ There are three types of elements of economics.

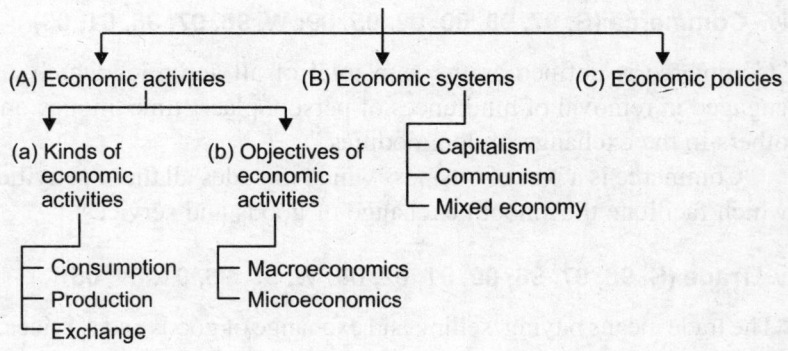

A. Economic Activities

They explain utilisation of natural and artificial sources.

(a) Kinds of Economic Activities

(i) **Consumption:** The activities undertaken to satisfy personal needs.

(ii) **Production:** It involves conversion of resources into finished products.

(iii) **Exchange:** The goods produced are exchanged to consumers.

(b) Objectives of Economic Activities

(i) **Macroeconomics:**
   I. National income
   II. Trade cycle
   III. Inflation
   IV. Financial institutions

(ii) **Microeconomics:** The points to be covered are:
   I. Theory of demands
   II. Theory of production
   III. Price determination
   IV. Product distribution

B. Economic Systems

Any country can adapt any suitable system for the economic development of the people in the country. These systems can be:

(i) Capitalism
(ii) Communism
(iii) Mixed economy

C. Economic Policies

Economic policies are problem-oriented. It is very common that "while solving any problem, other problems arise".

The government desides policies about various problems like:

• Population size
• Education
• Employment
• Health

4 Define industry. Classify industry/types of industry. (S. 06; W. 04, 05)

☞ **Industry**

"Industry is a part of business activity which is related to activities like production, repacking, extraction, fabrication, manufacturing, processing, etc."

Classification of Industry

A. Classification as per Nature of the Industry

1. *Genetic industry:* It undertakes growth and sale of plants and animals, e.g. nurseries and poultries.

2. *Extractive industry:* It undertakes extraction of soil or other parts of nature, e.g. mines, fisheries.

3. *Construction industry:* It undertakes construction of roads, damps, houses, rails, ports, etc.

4. *Manufacturing industry:* It undertakes manufacturing.

   (a) Analytical industry, e.g. petroleum products industry.

   (b) Assembling industry, e.g. autoindustry, computer industry.

   (c) Synthetic industry, e.g. chemical industry, cement industry.

   (d) Processing industry, e.g. sugar industry, textile industry.

B. Classification as per Capital Investment

1. *Light industry/small scale industry:* The capital required is less, i.e. less than 2 crore. Production quantity is lesser. Effectivity is spread over lesser geographical area.

2. *Heavy industry/large scale industry:* The capital required is tremendous, i.e. more than 2 crore. Production quantity is larger. Effectivity is spread over larger geographical area.

5 Define 'trade'. Classify trade. Give types or categories of trade. (S. 96, 97, 98, 00, 01, 02, 03, 06; W. 97, 99, 01, 04, 05)

☞ **Trade**

"The trade means buying, selling and exchange of goods and services."

Classification of Trade

A. As per Size of Trade

1. *Wholesale trade:* Trade quantity is larger.
2. *Retail sale trade:* Trade quantity is smaller.

B. As per Geographical Area

1. *Home trade:* When trading appears within a border of single country, it is known as home trade.
   (i) *Local trade:* Purchase and sale take place in one district.
   (ii) *State trade:* Purchase and sale take place in the state.
   (iii) *Interstate trade:* Purchase and sale take place in between the states.
2. *Foreign trade/international trade:* When two or more countries are involved in trading, it is known as foreign trade.
   . (i) *Import trade:* Import of material from foreign country.
   (ii) *Export trade:* Export of material to foreign country.
   (iii) *Entrepot trade:* The import and export take place within the involvement of another country.

6 Define 'aids to trade'. Explain various 'aids to trade'. Describe in brief auxiliaries to trade. (S. 00, 01, 02, 04, 05, 06, 07, 08, 09; W. 98, 06)

☞ Aids to Trade

"The factors which remove hindrances in trading are known as aids to trade."

Various aids to trade are:

1. Transport

- Transport is a medium which takes the product from one place to another.
- It makes the products available in retail stores and it provides more space for storage of products in industry and at wholesalers. Thus, transport removes hindrance of place.

2. Warehousing (Storage)

- It is the duty of producer or supplier to make the product available whenever required.

- Warehousing promotes the trade by saving time and so warehousing removes hindrance of time.

3. Banking and Finance

- Bank and other institutions provide money to manufacturers, traders and individual persons.
- So, banking removes hindrance of money.

4. Insurance

- Insurance covers losses due to earthquake, fire, flood, thefts, etc.
- So, insurance removes hindrance of risk.

5. Advertising and Salesmanship

- Both inform the public about availability of product and qualities of product.
- So, advertising and salesmanship remove the hindrance of knowledge.

6. Packaging

- Packaging removes hindrance of spoilage of goods.

7. Trade as Aid to Trade

- The product travels from manufacturer to customer through a channel.
- Wholesaler purchases product from manufacturer and sells to retailers.
- A retailer purchases product from wholesaler and sells to customers. These steps promote entire trade.
- Thus, trade itself is one of the aids to trade.

7 Define management. Describe functions of management/pharmaceutical management. (S. 98, 99, 02, 04, 05, 06, 07, 09; W. 96, 97, 98, 99, 02, 03, 06, 07)

☞ Management

"Management is a distinct process consisting of planning, organising, activating and controlling all operations to determine and fulfill the objectives of organisation."

Functions of Management

A. Primary Functions

1. **Planning**
   - It is the most fundamental function of management.
   - It is based upon past events, needs and objectives.
   - For better planning, the managers should have a vision of future.
   - The managers should sit together and exchange their ideas about the past and future.
   - Managers determine course of action to be taken only after analysing situation.
   - The managers determine primary goals and targets and policies along with secondary goals and targets and policies.
   - Planning is necessary to achieve better results.
   - Proper planning involves full production, inventory control and sales organisation.

2. **Organising**
   - The management should form various departments and responsibilities are given to the people of related departments.
   - The departments should be interlinked with each other.

3. **Staffing**
   - A right person should be selected for a right job.
   - The duties and powers of the person appointed should be well defined.
   - Staffing pattern should be as per qualifications and experience.
   - Staffing should be done as per requirement and compensation may be given according to performance.

4. **Motivating**
   - Motivation or inspiration is to promote the staff.
   - Guide the staff in positive direction.
   - Motivation can be achieved by offering freedom of expression, job expansion and award.
   - It creates harmony in organisation.

5. **Coordinating**
   - Coordination of various departments is necessary for effective functioning of organisation.

- Various activities should be streamlined.
- It helps to solve the problem, exchange of ideas of both the persons and the departments.

6. **Controlling**
   - Controlling involves day-to-day observations in working.
   - Lower performance of workers without suitable reason is never tolerated by management.
   - Strong controls are more harmful than very loose control.
   - Management calculates the average of controls after analysing performance and reasons for failure.

7. **Directing**
   - In order to complete the goals and targets, each higher level manager should give proper directions to lower persons.
   - Directing can be done by training, ordering, instructing, demonstrating and counselling.

B. **Secondary Functions:**

1. **Communication**
   - Management should have good communication with staff and workers.
   - Management should provide common platform to the staff to express their feelings, freely emotions, facts and ideas about the organisation.

2. **Innovation**
   - It is a continuous process of taking care of technological developments and lifestyle of workers.
   - Management should use intraprofessional information to minimise the strain or stress and improve job satisfaction.

Forms of Business Organisation

1 **What are the characteristics of an ideal form of business organisation?**

☞ The ideal form of business organisation should possess:
1. Ease of formation.
2. Ease of raising finance or capital.
3. Limited liability.
4. Flexibility of operation.
5. Stability or continuity.
6. Retention of business secrete.
7. Freedom from state regulations.
8. Lower tax liability.

2 **What are the factors affecting selection of business form?**

☞ The following factors affect (influence) the selection of business form:
1. Scope, size and life of business.
2. Ease in formation.
3. Risk
4. Flexibility.
5. Government policies, controls of taxation.
6. Business secretes.
7. Area of operation.
8. Nature of goods to be produced.

9. Requirement of finance and sources available.
10. Liability aspects.

3 **State/classify different forms of business organi-sation. (S. 96, 97, 00, 03; W. 96, 97, 98, 00)**

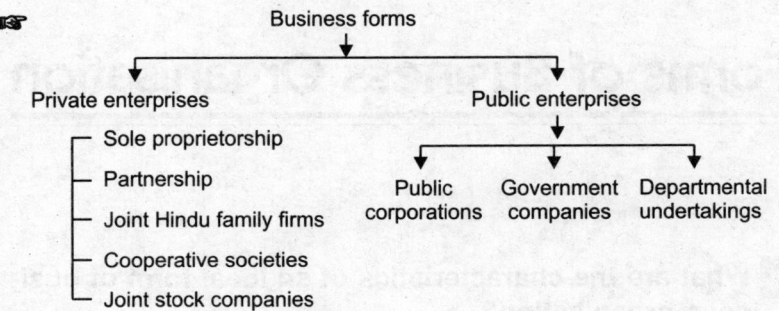

4 **What is sole proprietorship? Give its features, advantages and disadvantages. (W. 97)**

☞ **Sole proprietorship**

"When business is owned by one person, it is known as sole proprietorship or sole tradership."

Features

1. Single ownership.
2. Common identity, i.e. owner and business are same.
3. Capital investment should be done by owner himself.
4. Liabilities are on the proprietors only.
5. Direct control of owner on all activities.
6. He is responsible for all profits or losses in the business.

Advantages

1. Profits are not shared with others.
2. Very easy to start or to dissolve.
3. Diversification of business is possible.
4. The business secrecy is the highest.
5. It offers a pleasure of decision-making.
6. Prompt decisions can be taken without consulting with others.
7. Customer-oriented service can be given.

8. Personal relations with customers can be maintained.
9. Minimum government regulations to sole tradership.
10. It generates self-employment on large scale.

Disadvantages

1. Limited finance is available hence less growth.
2. Limited activities, limited customers, so limited sales and comparatively less profits.
3. Losses and liabilities are not shared and increased risk.
4. Possibility of taking wrong decisions.
5. Difficult to develop market and create goodwill of business.
6. The owner has to depend upon others in the field of government policies, taxation and legal matters.
7. The death of the owner may put full stop of the business.
8. Impact in limited geographical area.

5 **Define partnership. Give features, advantages and disadvantages of partnership. (S. 96, 98, 00, 01, 03; W. 96, 97, 98, 01, 07, 08)**

☞ **Partnership**

"A partnership is a form of business organisation in which two or more persons carry business together for the purpose of earning profits."

Features/Characteristics

1. There should be minimum 2 and maximum 20 persons in business.
2. Partnership firm is created by an agreement under Partnership Act.
3. Partners share in both profit and losses.
4. Every partner is entitled to take part in management of day-to-day work.
5. All the partners are liable jointly for all debts of the firm.

Advantages

1. There is an availability of more capital, so more is the size of business and profit.
2. Life of business is more.

3. There is a less possibility to take wrong decision, due to presence of other partners.
4. Better management is possible.
5. The registration procedures and legal formalities are easier.
6. Financial results need not be declared to the customers.
7. Quick decision-making can be possible by coming together of all parners.
8. It can maintain better human public relations.
9. In partnership firm, partners are flexible to start new business jointly whenever they desire.

Disadvantages

1. Retirement or death of active partner may end the business.
2. Personal ambitions of any partner may bring the business in danger.
3. It is difficult to maintain positive relationship in all the partners for a long time.
4. Less secracy.
5. Lack of public confindence.
6. Unlimited liability.

6 **Write a note on "partnership deed" or describe in brief the formation and agreement of partnership deed. (S. 98, 06, 07)**

☞ **Partnership Deed**

The document containing agreement with partners in partnership business is known as partnership deed.

(a) Agreement between the partners is done by an agreement on stamp papers. This document is known as partnership deed.
(b) The terms and conditions are known as articles and should include the following points:
    1. Name and address of organisation.
    2. Nature and duration of business.
    3. Capital to be invested.
    4. Names of all partners.
    5. Addresses of all partners.
    6. Dates of birth of all partners.
    7. Other occupations of all partners and professional addresses.

8. Share of each partner in capital, profit and loss.
9. Other responsibilities of each partner in business.
10. Mode of repayment of the capital and rate of interest on it.
11. Maximum amount of money that can be withdrawn by any partner at a time and rate of interest on it.
12. Other benefits for partners.
13. Terms and conditions for inclusion, exclusion or retirement of new or present partners.
14. Dissolution of the firm.
15. Salary or remuneration or commission of the partners.

7 **Explain different kinds/types of partners in partnership business. (S. 97, 98, 00, 04, 05, 06, 09; W. 98, 03, 04)**

☞ **Types of Partners**

(a) Active or acting partner:
- He takes active part in routine of business.
- He is also known as working partner.
- He takes all decisions about the business and others are supposed to agree with decision taken by active partner.

(b) Passive/dormant/sleeping partner: He shares in capital, profit and loss but do not take active part in the business.

(c) Nominal partner:
- A nominal partner allows his name to be used in title of organisation.
- He is legally responsible for the business activities.
- He does not contribute in capital, profit and losses.

(d) Secrete partner: His name is not disclosed to outsiders like bankers, suppliers or customers.

(e) Minor as a partner:
- Actually minor cannot be partner of any business.
- In some countries like USA, a minor can share in capital, profit and losses.

(f) Partners in profit only: He shares in profit only.

(g) Subpartner: Partner of the firm agrees to share his own share of the firm with an outsider such a partner is known as sub-partner.

(h) Silent partner: He has no voice in management but he shares profit and losses of the firm.

(i) **Partners on holding out.**

(j) **Partner by estoppel.**

8 **What is Joint Hindu Family firm? Give its features, advantages and disadvantages. (S. 98, 99, 03, 05, 06, 07; W. 05)**

☞ **Joint Hindu Family Firm**

"It is a distinct form of business organisation, which is governed by Hindu laws and customs."

Features/Characteristics

1. Only male persons can be members or owner of the business.
2. From the birth in the family he becomes the member of the firm.
3. Minor can be the owner of the firm.
4. The head of the family is *karta* and he has all rights to manage the business and take decision.
5. The shares in profit and other benefits to other family members are determined by the owner.
6. The other family members do not share in liabilities.
7. Termination of the business is possible only when the male line in the family discontinues.

Advantages

1. The business continues for several generations.
2. *Karta* has full powers to run the business without interference by any other member.
3. Cooperative efforts of all the members of the family can make the business more prosperous.
4. Social status to the business, to the owner and to the members in observed.
5. Other members have limited liability.

Disadvantages

1. It is difficult to motivate other family members in business activities.
2. There may be injustice in some members of family.
3. Continuity of male line succession in the family is very important.

4. Diversification of business is not possible.
5. Incapable head of the family may bring the business in danger.
6. Small family quarrels may reduce growth of business.
7. Limited resources.

9 **What do you mean by cooperative form of business organisation? Give features, advantages and disadvantages. (S. 96, 98, 00, 02, 05, 06, 08; W. 03, 04, 06)**

☞ **Definition**

"Cooperative organisation is an association of persons usually of limited means, who voluntarily joined together to achieve a common economic end and promotion of economic interest of its members in accordance with cooperative principles."

Features

1. Association of persons: Membership is open to all.
2. Voluntary membership: No compulsion for joining or leaving.
3. Common economic end.
4. Democratic control: It is run as per democratic principles.
5. Contribution to capital: Every member has to contribute to capital before joining the group.
6. Benefits and risk: Profits and losses are equally distributed depending upon the share.
7. Registration: It should be registered under Indian Cooperative Society Act, 1912.
8. Trading: The cooperative organisation trade on cash basis only.
9. Motive: The motive is not to earn large profits but to give services to society.

Advantages

1. This form is most suitable for a common man.
2. It is very easy to get the membership of cooperative organisation.
3. Living in group is also possible.
4. There is a whole-hearted support from government to this form. The support may be in terms of less taxation or loose government controls.
5. For a member risks and liabilities are very limited.
6. It generates large scale employment.

Disadvantages

1. The field of functioning is limited.
2. There is no scope for expansion or bringing flexibility in business.
3. Inefficient management is a common drawback.
4. Secrecy cannot be maintained.
5. The impact spreads in comparatively less geographical area.
6. Every possible disadvantage of democratic functioning.
7. Changes in government policies can bring the business in problem.

10 **What do you understand by "joint stock company"? Give features, advantages and disadvantages. (S. 07, 09; W. 03, 05)**

☞ **Definition**

"Joint stock company is an organisation of individuals for earning profit in which capital is divided into transferable shares."

Features

1. **Artificial person:** Organisation can enter in contract just like a single person.
2. **Membership is voluntary:** Shares are transferable. Entry and leaving of membership is not binding.
3. Value of shares is fixed throughout the life of business.
4. Profits and liabilities of a shareholder are in the proportion of his investment.
5. **Registration:** The company should be registered as per Indian Company Law.
6. Retirement or death of single or some shareholders has no effect on company.
7. **A common seal:** A common seal is to be prepared to make documents valid. It is used by official persons only.
8. **Separation of ownership and management:** Shareholders have no right to participate in day-to-day activities.
9. The company undertakes business as mentioned in "Memorandum of Association."

Advantages

1. Maximum capital is available.
2. Liabilities of shareholders are minimum.

3. Life of business is more.
4. It generates large scale employment.
5. Share can be transferred.
6. Business has skilled management.
7. Democratic functioning.
8. For government, the companies are good sources of tax collection.

Disadvantages

1. Difficult in formation.
2. Lack of working in managers brings the business in danger.
3. No quick decision can be taken.
4. Possibility of misappropriation and frauds.
5. No secrecy.
6. Government monitors activities keenly.

11 **Differentiate between private and public limited companies.**

☞

Private limited companies	Public limited companies
1. Number of members 2 to 50	1. Minimum 7 members
2. Share transfers are more restricted	2. Share transfers less restricted
3. Number of directors are minimum two	3. Number of directors minimum three
4. Allotment to new shares to any person	4. Preference share is given to existing shareholder
5. Title—XYZ Pvt. Ltd.	5. Title—ABC Ltd.

12 **What do you mean by government enterprises/public enterprises/state enterprises?**

☞ **Public Enterprises**

• These are owned by state or central government.
• Their aim is to promote industrial and economical development on large scale.

Definition

Public enterprises means ownership in operation of industrial agricultural, financial and commercial undertaking.

Features

1. Entire finance/capital is provided by government.
2. They are owned by government.
3. The objective is to provide service to the citizens.
4. The government is answerable about these activities in the "Houses of Parliament".
5. In some areas entry of private sectors is totally prohibited, it generates monopoly of the government.

Objectives

1. To have balanced economic growth in the country.
2. To generate employment on large scale.
3. To promote industrialisation in the areas where capital requirement is beyond calculation.
4. To avoid exploitation of the society from private sector.
5. To impliment effectively the government policies.
6. To increase state revenues.
7. For the safety of the people, government has to enter in some areas.

13 Differentiate between (a) sole tradership/proprietorship and partnership, (b) partnership and joint Hindu family.

☞ **(a) Sole Tradership/Proprietorship and Partnership (S. 06)**

Features	Sole tradership/ proprietorship	Partnership
1. Secrecy	More	Less
2. Life	Less	More
3. Profit amount	Lesser	More
4. Capital	Less	More
5. Act	No Act	Indian Partnership Act
6. Number of owners	Himself (one)	2 to 20
7. Owner is	Proprietor	Partner
8. Source	Only one	Share in partners
9. Stability of business	Low	High
10. Management	Depends upon knowledge of owner	Management is better

(b) Partnership and Joint Hindu Family

Features	Partnership	Joint Hindu family
1. Origin	Formed by agreement	By birth in the family
2. Number of members	2 to 20	No limit
3. Male/female	Female can be partner	Female cannot be member
4. Minor	Minor cannot be a partner but avail benefit	A male member becomes member by birth in the family
5. Liability	The liabilities of the partners are unlimited	The liability of *karta* is unlimited
6. Law	Indian Partnership Act 1932 is applicable	Hindu laws and customs are applicable
7. Participation in business	All partners have equal rights to take part in business	Only *karta* can manage the business
8. Agency relationship	Every partner is an agent	Only *karta* is empowered as agent
9. Death or insolvency	A firm dissolves by death or insolvency of a *karta*	A joint Hindu family is dissolved by the death of a *karta*

Channels of Distribution

1 Define "channels of distribution". Give advantages of channels of distribution. (S. 98, 00, 04; W. 03)

☞ **Channels of Distribution**

"The channels of distribution are the routes by which the goods are moved from the producer to the ultimate customer."

Advantages

1. The goods are easily available at all the places.
2. The financial burden is very less due to channels of distribution.
3. The sale of goods increase due to support of wholesaler and retailers.
4. The goods are available at similar prices throughout the area.
5. It gives more employment.
6. It allows distribution of goods in small quantity.
7. The goods are available in remote area also.
8. The cost of marketing is reduced by channels of distribution.

2 Define 'market' and 'pharmaceutical market'. What do you mean by direct and indirect market in pharmaceutical market?

☞ **a. Market**

"Market is the geographical place where purchaser and seller come in personal contact."

b. Pharmaceutical Market

"The pharmaceutical market is the market of every specialized product like medicaments, drugs, cosmetics, toilet preparations and other similar products." It is categorised into:

i. Direct Market

In this process, the customer is allowed to select the product of his choice and the products can be purchased without consulting experts, e.g. OTC products, and analgesics, antitussives, expectorants, toilet preparations.

ii. Indirect Market

The customer has to follow the order of physician (prescription), e.g. antibiotics, antidiabetics, antimalarials.

3 Enlist different channels of distribution for general and pharmaceutical products.

☞ (A) General Products

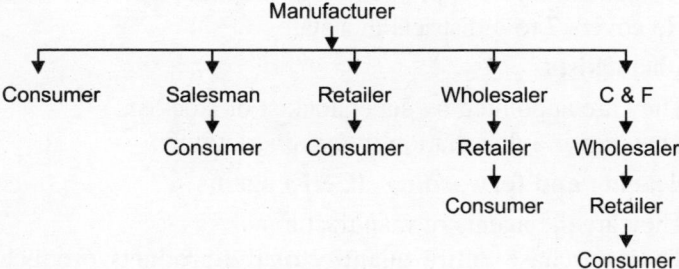

(B) Pharmaceutical Products (S. 04)

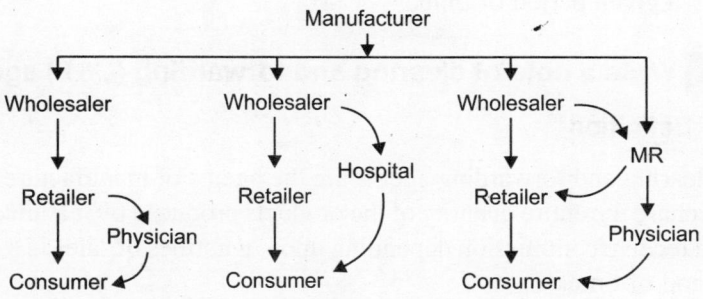

4 Define wholesalers. Explain types of wholesalers. (S. 06)

☞ **Wholesalers**

"Wholesalers are the traders who purchase the products in bulk from the manufacturer and sale them to retailers or consumers."

Types of Wholesalers

(a) Superstockist	(1 to 2 states)
(b) Stockist	(2 to 4 districts)
(c) Substockist	(1 district)
(d) Clearing and forwarding agents	(C and F)

(a) Superstockist

- A superstockist is appointed by manufacturer.
- He covers larger geographical area, i.e. in one or two states.
- He has to purchase the products in large quantities.
- He has to store the products properly to satisfy the market needs of the entire area.

(b) Stockist

- A stockist may be appointed by the manufacturer or wholesaler.
- He covers 2 to 4 districts in a state.

(c) Substockists

- They are appointed by superstockist or stockist.
- They cover a distribution in one district only.

(d) Clearing and forwarding (C&F) agents

- They are the agents of manufacturer.
- They purchase entire quantity of the products produced by manufacturer.
- They receive commission depending upon quantities of sales in a given period of time.

5 Write a note of clearing and forwarding (C&F) agents.

☞ **Definition**

"Clearing and forwarding agents are the agents of manufacturer who purchase the entire quantity of the products produced by manufacturer and receive commission depending upon quantities of sales in a given period of time."

Reasons/Need for Appointing C&F Agent

1. Manufacturer wants to avoid its entry in marketing and wants to concentrate on manufacturing activities.
2. The manufacturer is lacking in the knowledge of market and marketing.
3. The manufacturer does not have suitable manpower for marketing.

Selection of C&F Agent

- The manufacturer selects C&F agent carefully.
- Manufacturer invites applications from proposed C&F agents.
- Manufacturer holds the discussion with applicants and may ask the C&F agent to deposit large amounts of money.
- The manufacturer confirms the documents enclosed with applications regarding:
    (i) Financial capacity
    (ii) Ability to handle manpower
    (iii) Availability of sufficient space for storage.
- The agent which fulfills above requirements is appointed as C&F agent.

Functions of C&F Agent

1. Proper storage of materials.
2. To maintain uniform flow of product in market.
3. Periodical reporting to manufacturer.
4. To maintain accounts.
5. To settle concerned taxes.

Expectations from C&F Agent

1. He should have sound financial position.
2. He should store the quantities of products and should provide a sufficient space.
3. He should provide proper storage conditions to the products, e.g. racks, shelves, refrigerators, air conditioning, etc.
4. He should appoint staff and marketing representatives.
5. The C&F is expected to look after well being of manpower.
6. He should market the products quickly.

7. He should forward the advertising materials prepared by manufacturers.
8. He should forward information booklets to the customers.
9. He should clear the credit given to customers.
10. He should settle the account of the purchase with the manufacturer.
11. He should inform the market trends to the manufacturer.
12. He should give advice to the manufacturer about taxation and government policies.

6 What are various functions/duties of wholesalers? (S. 98, 02, 03, 08, 09; W. 98, 06)

☞ 1. To purchase the products in large quantities from different manufacturers.
2. To store the products at proper storage conditions.
3. Grading and standardisation of goods.
4. Assembling of goods in a good fashion.
5. Attaching information booklets, free gifts with the products.
6. Suitable packaging of products.
7. Forwarding discount and other schemes to the customers.
8. Offering credit to the customers.
9. To transport the goods from factories and supply to retailers.
10. To provide market information regarding products and sale to the manufacturer.
11. The certain types of goods (except drugs), prices are fixed by the wholesaler himself.

7 Give the advantages and disadvantages of wholesale trade/wholesalers. (S. 01, 02; W. 02, 07)

☞ **Advantages/Merits/Services of Wholesalers**

(a) To Producer or Manufacturer

1. They provide information regarding market.
2. They help in advertisement of products.
3. They provide financial help by giving advances.
4. They help in supply of drugs to small areas.
5. Due to advance orders, production can be done at large scale.

(b) To Retailers

1. Medicines of different manufacturers are available at one place.
2. Medicines can be purchased in very small quantities by retailers.
3. They provide credit facilities to retailers.
4. They provide the information regarding change in prices.
5. They adjust the expiry and breakage of medicines.
6. They provide discount on bulk or cash purchase.
7. They also supply the medicines to retailers by their own vehicle.

Disadvantages/Demerits of Wholesalers

1. They increase the price of goods by increasing their margin of profit.
2. Wholesale of drugs and medicines should be done under Drugs and Cosmetics Act, 1940.
3. Sometimes, they do not supply in time.
4. They create an artificial shortage of stock by depositing large amount of goods in secrete place.

8 Define retailers. Give the functions/importance of retailers. (S. 01, 06, 09; W. 03)

☞ **Retailers**

Retailers are the traders who purchase the product from wholesalers comparatively in smaller quantities and sell them to customers.

Functions/Importance of Retailers

1. To make available wide range of products to satisfy needs of society.
2. To store the products in proper storage conditions.
3. Assembling the products.
4. Gradation and standardisation of products.
5. To handover the product to the customer which may satisfy the need of customer.
6. To provide credit facilities to their regular customers.
7. To offer customer-oriented service.
8. To help the manufacturer in introducing new product in the market.

9. To promote OTC sale.
10. To provide a proper information for market research.
11. To arrange attractive display in show windows and promote sale of goods.
12. To bear the risk of fire, theft, bad debts, etc.
13. They help in rapid distribution of production.
14. Retailers reduce transaction between manufacturer and customer.
15. As retailers are in very large number, they strengthen and diffuse the economy.

9 **Mention the advantages of retailers. OR What services are given by the retailer to manufacturer and wholesaler? (S. 01; W. 03)**

☞ **Advantages of Retailers to Manufacturer and Wholesalers**

1. They are the important link between manufacturer and customer.
2. They provide feedback information.
3. Sometimes, they make advance payment and give financial facilities.
4. They make advertisement and window displays of the products.
5. They provide information necessary for market research.
6. The retailers also provide information regarding customers' likings, preference and change of design of the product.

10 **Explain the role of retailers in pharmacy.**

☞ In pharmacy field, the retailers work as either:
 (i) Hospital pharmacist or
 (ii) Community pharmacist
The community pharmacists are more important than hospital pharmacists, because they market the products to the large section of society. They are known as "chemists and druggists".
The persons working in these retailing should be registered pharmacists (having diploma/degree in pharmacy) and help:
 1. To maintain adequate stock of large varieties of drugs/medicines.
 2. To make available similar products manufactured by various manufacturers.

3. To check authenticity of the prescription.
4. To inform the patient about the product.

Duties of Retailers

1. He should do proper patient counselling.
2. He should clarify the doubts in Rx and dispense the dosage accurately.
3. He should promote OTC sale.
4. He should record the changes in improvement in patient.

11 **What do you understand by departmental stores? Give features, advantages and disadvantages of departmental store. (S. 00, 02, 05, 07; W. 97, 98, 99)**

☞ **Departmental Store**

"A departmental store is a big store engaged in a retail trade of wide variety of products under the same roof."

Features

1. In a departmental store, retail business is carried out on large scale.
2. All departments work under the same roof.
3. Each department markets particular range of products.
4. Centralized purchasing procedure is followed.
5. It involves marketing of all types of products from consumer goods to luxurious goods.
6. It requires huge capital investment.
7. Its location should be near to the central place in the city.
8. It undertakes the sales in cash basis only.
9. Cost of running is very high.
10. It gives pleasure in purchasing by allowing product handling, demonstration and by offering facilities like garden, restaurants.

Advantages

1. A customer gets a wide choice of products.
2. The customer has pleasure and satisfaction in purchase process.
3. Customers can purchase all items at one place.
4. A customer is allowed to handle the products.
5. Prices of the product are fixed, there is no bargaining.

6. Customers get services of trained manpower.
7. It is good site for advertisement.
8. Ensures good quality of product.
9. Due to large turnover, the margin of profit is much higher.
10. Loss of a department can be covered by profit from other departments.

Disadvantages

1. Heavy capital investment.
2. Cost of running is very high.
3. The prices of products are higher.
4. There are chances of misuse of other facilities provided to customers.
5. Difficult to manage activities of all departments.
6. Lack of personal motivation in workers.
7. They undertake sale in cash basis only.

12 Define 'multiple shop'/chain shop. Give features, merits, and demerits. (S. 00, 04, 05, 07; W. 05)

☞ **Multiple Shop**

"It is a system of branch shops operated under centralized management and dealing in limited range of products."

Features

1. Multiple shop sells goods of one manufacturer only.
2. The products in limited range are marketed.
3. The products marketed are generally essential consumer goods.
4. The purchasing is centralized.
5. Layout design, decoration and colour scheme of all shops are same.
6. They are located at the corners of a city.
7. Sales are in cash basis only.
8. There is a high flexibility in opening new branches and closing the existing branches.
9. Advertisement for all shops remains the same.
10. It eliminates both wholesaler and retailer.

Advantages

1. No bargaining is allowed as prices are fixed.
2. Quality of goods is better.
3. Reasonable prices of the products.
4. Comparatively lesser cost of running.
5. Due to centralized purchase, finance required for purchasing is reduced.
6. A branch in poor condition of sale can be easily closed.
7. Centralized advertisement increases sales of all shops.
8. Total cash business provides no bad debt.
9. Loss of a branch can be covered by profit from other branches.
10. Generally, layout design of all shops is same, which creates a special image and status of the shop.

Disadvantages

1. Capital investment is very high.
2. If offers no credit facility.
3. Lack of personal motivation in workers.
4. Difficulties in centralized control and management.
5. The system offers only limited range of products.
6. Not suitable for pharmaceutical formulations.

13 What is mail order business? Give its features, advantages and disadvantages. (S. 08, W. 97, 04, 06)

☞ **Mail order Business**

"It is a kind of retail trade which receives order by post and deliver the articles by post."

Features

1. There is no necessity of establishment of a formal shop.
2. The products which are having light weights and are unbreakable can only be marketed.
3. Role of advertisement like catalogue, leaflets, newspapers is very important.

Advantages

1. Goods are received at door itself.
2. Less capital is required.

3. Cost of running is less.
4. The products can be distributed in any corner of the world.
5. Physical efforts of customers are saved.
6. Goods are sent by VPP and thus chances of bad debts are negligible.
7. There is no middleman.
8. The business is regular and production can be done after receiving orders.
9. Overhead expenses are not required and thus very economical.

Disadvantages

1. There is a lack of personal contact.
2. Postal delay causes inconvenience.
3. Frauds can be done with innocent customers.
4. No after sales service is provided.
5. No credit facility is available.
6. Possibility of breakage during VPP (Value Payable Post).
7. Goods are costlier because of post expenses.
8. The system is unsuitable for all types of goods.
9. Scope of business is limited to educated persons only.
10. The cost of advertisement is higher.
11. The time period in the process is more.

14 Explain types of mail order business.

☞ There are three main types of mail order business:

(i) Manufacturer Mail Order House

These are established by the manufacturers for selling the goods manufactured by them directly to the consumers, thus eliminating middleman.

(ii) Departmental Mail Order Business

This is only a department of a departmental store executing orders received from outside.

(iii) Middleman Mail Order Business

In this case the business house is not engaged in production or wholesale selling but concerned only with the sale of goods by mail.

It purchases the required goods, partly on the receipt of orders and partly in anticipation of orders, from the wholesaler and despatches the same by mail to the consumers.

15 **Differentiate between departmental stores and multiple shop. (S. 03; W. 04)**

☞

No.	Basis	Departmental store	Multiple shop
1.	Variety of products	Wide variety of products to satisfy all types of requirements	Products of only one manufacturer
2.	Price	Prices are more	Prices are minimum
3.	Location	It should be located at heart of cities	It can be situated at any place
4.	Services	It gives personal services to customers	It does not give personal services to customers
5.	Credit	They give credit to their regular customers	They do not give credit
6.	Risk	They have great risk as their working place is fixed	They have less risk because they can change the place of shop
7.	Advertisement	Local advertisement	Nationwide advertisement
8.	Capital required	Capital investment is very high	Comparatively low capital investment
9.	Facilities provided to customers	Facilities like garden, restaurant are provided	No facilities are provided

16 **What do you understand by "hire purchase trading system?" Mention its advantages and disadvantages. (S. 96. 06)**

☞ **Hire Purchase Trading System**

It is the system of purchasing the goods in which purchaser gets the possession of goods without paying the full amount to seller.

- A part of payment is made at the time of purchase and rest in installments.

- In this system buyer becomes the owner of the goods only after payment of total price.
- If the purchaser does not pay installment, the seller is free to carry back the goods.
- This whole system works on an agreement signed between the seller and the buyer with or without guarantor.
- Hire purchase system is usually carried in case of durable consumer articles like cars, radios, televisions, coolers, refrigerators.

Advantages

1. It is the best way to buy certain valuable articles without payment of full value.
2. The small and medium scale manufacturers increase their sell by this system.
3. Increase the turnover of nonessential luxury articles.
4. Interest charge is lower than the bank interest.

Disadvantages

1. People may buy things which they cannot afford.
2. It makes article costlier.
3. The traders run a very heavy risk.

Drug House Management

1 **How will you select a site to open a new medical store/ shop? OR What factors are to be considered during selection of site for new drug store? (S. 01, 02, 05, 07, 08; W. 96, 98, 06)**

Selection of Site

☞ The following factors should be considered while selecting a site for new drug store:
  A. Rural area
  B. Urban area
  C. Other factors
    • Number of physicians
    • Number of hospitals
    • Presence of other drug store
    • Traffic
    • Residential areas
    • Gathering places
    • Business locality
    • Developing areas
    • Lifestyle of customers

A. Rural Area

In village, the population is less and awareness in society about health is less. It results in less number of physicians. The people in villages have less buying capacity because of less finance. The medical store requires less investment. The prescription sales are less and sales of OTC products is more.

B. Urban Area

In urban area population is more and awareness in society about health is more. It results in large number of physicians. The people in urban areas have more buying capacity because of more availability of finance.

In drug store, prescription sale is more and sale of OTC product is less in comparision with rural areas.

The medical stores in urban areas should be attractive and thus cost of running is more. But due to high margin of profit and sale, urban areas are the good sites for opening new drug stores.

C. Other Factors

1. *Number of physicians:* The area where 3 to 4 physicians are consulting, it is the best site for opening new drug store and business will be good.
2. *Number of hospitals:* One or two hospitals near the area of drug store make the business in good manner.
3. *Presence of other drug store:*
   - Ideally there should not be any competition, but if potential of the area is high, then 2 to 3 drug stores in the same area can be survived.
   - If reputation of existing store is poor, the place is open to all.
4. *Traffic:*
   - Heavy traffic of vehicles is not a good site for business.
   - Drug stores near the signals, one way roads should be avoided.
   - More the traffic of persons, more is the business.
5. *Residential areas:*
   - The places at the centre of residential area are ideal sites.
   - In these cases, Rx sales and OTC sales both are maximum.
6. *Gathering places:* The places like school, colleges, cinema hall, theatres, market places, large government offices are good sites.
7. *Business locality:* The drug stores in commercial areas require heavy investment.
8. *Developing areas:* Developing areas are the good sites.
9. *Lifestyle of customers:* It is essential to maintain stock of drug, availability of variety and to make the attractive design of the store.

2 Write a note on "acquisition of premise."

☞ **Acquisition of Premise**

- Once the site is selected the businessman has to acquire it.
- There are two modes of acquisition:

A. Outright Purchase

- It is beneficial in long time run.
- It requires huge amount of money.
- Owner has to develop and provide all facilities.

B. Rental Basis

1. The owner accepts any person as a user and user has to pay some cash to landlord which is the rent.
2. The owner should be bound to provide some facilities to the user.
3. There is an agreement or lease between the owner and user.
4. The lease or agreement should contain following points:
   - Name and address of owner (landlord).
   - Name and address of user (tenant).
   - Name and address of the place to be rented.
   - Nature of the business.
   - Amount of rent.
   - Mode of payment of rent.
   - Duration of agreement.
   - Responsibility of landlord.
   - Responsibility of user.
   - Signatures of landlord and tenant.
   - If anyone fails in performing responsibilities, agreement can be cancelled.
   - Misuse of premise by any party may results in cancellation of agreement.

3 Define "layout design" of drug store. Give objectives of layout design. (S. 97, 98, 99, 00, 07)

☞ **Layout Design**

Definition

The layout design is the plan explaining proper and maximum utilisation of space inside the four walls of business.

Requirements/Points Considered during Layout Design

• There should be signal entrance for the customers.
• The shop area should be separated from private rooms.
• The licence should be displayed prominently.
• Name of the shop should be easily readable.

Objectives of Layout Design

1. To attract the customers and to increase the sales.
2. To build up professional image.
3. Maximum utilization of space.
4. To control the traffic of customers.
5. To provide a sufficient space for salesman, additional stock, waste material and for rest.
6. To minimise number of persons working behind the counter.
7. To avoid thefts.
8. To satisfy the customers.

4 **Draw the layout of (a) retail drug store (b) wholesale drug store.**

☞ **(a) Layout of Retail Drug Store (S. 97, 98, 99, 00, 04, 05, 06, 09; W. 03, 04)**

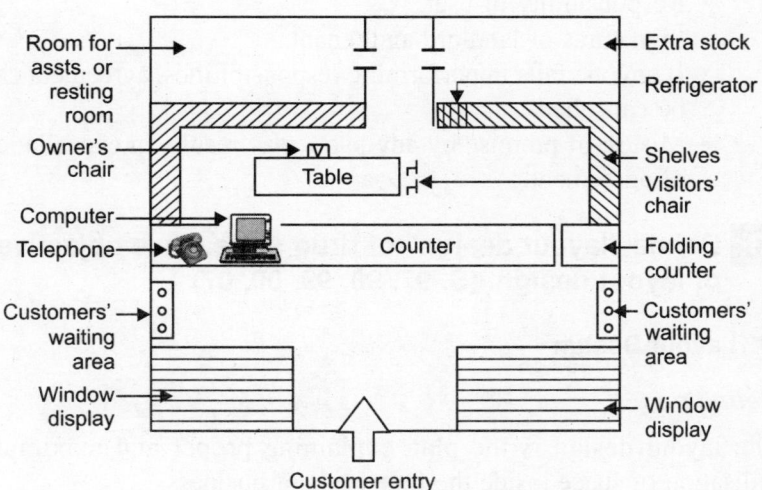

Customer entry

(b) Layout of Wholesale Drug Store (S. 99)

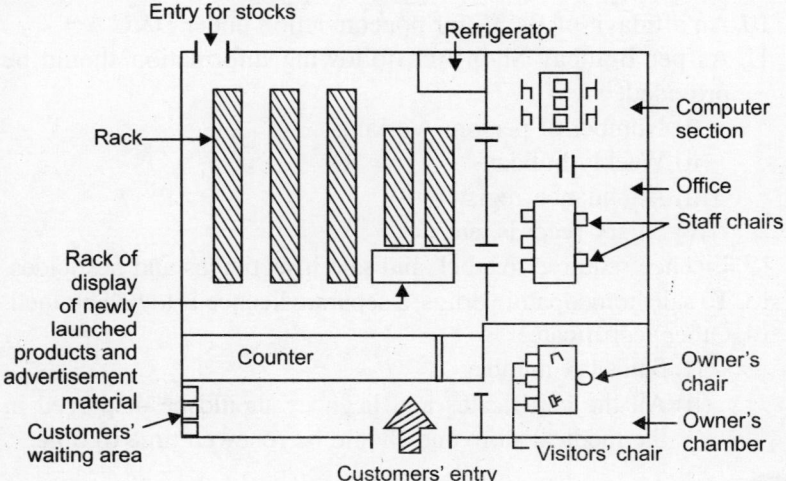

5 **What are the documents required for opening a new retail drug store? OR Enlist legal requirement and documents and licences required to open a new medical store. (S. 98, 01, 03, 05, 06, 09; W. 98, 99, 00, 01, 02, 04, 06)**

☞ 1. Application in duplicate in Form No. 19 B.
2. One copy for biological products and another copy for non-biological products.
3. A fee of Rs 200/- to be deposited in government treasury office along with Form No. 32 A.
4. Academic record:
  (a) Attested copy of mark list of diploma in pharmacy from institute approved by PCI (Ist and IInd yrs.)
  (b) Attested copy of registration certificate issued by state pharmacy council.
  (c) Affidavit of qualified person if the qualified person is an employee of the firm.
  (d) An attested copy of matriculation certificate for proof of birth date.
5. A plan or map of the premise.
6. Site or location of the premise.
7. Receipt of rents if the place is rented.

8. A copy of partnership deed if applicable.
9. A receipt showing purchase of refrigerator.
10. An affidavit of Rs 3/- for nonconviction under D&C Act.
11. As per Bombay Shop Act, following information should be provided:
    (i) Number of persons working
    (ii) Weekly holiday
    (iii) Attendance register
    (iv) Salary records, etc.
12. Licence required to stock and sale insecticides and pesticides.
13. To sale homeopathic drugs, a separate licence is to be obtained.
14. Other certificates:
    (i) Sales tax number
    (ii) All the certificates and licences should be displayed in the medical store and should be renewed time to time.

6 **What are legal requirements and documents required for new wholesale licence?**

☞ 1. Application in duplicate in Form No. 19.
2. One copy for biological and other copy for nonbiological products.
3. A fee of Rs 400/- should be deposited in government treasury office.
4. Attested copy of matriculation certificate.
5. Attested copy of experience certificate or attested copy of diploma in pharmacy.
6. Plan of premises.
7. Site of premises.
8. Copy of agreement if business is in partnership.
9. Receipt of purchase of refrigerator.
10. For schedule C and C_1 drugs, application should be submitted in Form No. 21 B.

7 **Define the terms—"purchase" and "purchasing". Give the objectives of purchasing. (S. 97, 98, 01, 02, 07, 08, 09; W. 96, 97, 99, 01, 06)**

☞ **Purchase**

"Purchase is the process of procurement of materials for the business to satisfy the business needs."

Purchasing

"Purchasing means the buying of right type of material in right quantity at the right time and at the right place."

Objectives of Purchasing

 (i) Right quality
 (ii) Right quantity
 (iii) Right source
 (iv) Right price
 (v) Right time
 (vi) Right place
 (vii) Right mode of transportation
 (viii) Right packaging

 (i) *Right quality:* The quality of the material is important in building reputation of business.

   Before placing any purchase order, a small quantity of product is obtained and quality is judged and then only final purchase order is placed.

 (ii) *Right quantity:* Many of the times the purchase quantity depends upon price structure, discounts, free gifts to attract the customers.

   Thus, the quantity purchased should not be excess than our requirement.

 (iii) *Right source:* The right source may be the manufacturer, C&F or authorised wholesaler.

   He should provide the materials continuously along with right quality.

 (iv) *Right price:* The price depends upon quality and quantity of the purchase material.

   Right price does not indicate the lowest price. The right quality with comparative minimum price is the right price.

 (v) *Right time:* The materials should be purchased as and when they are required to maintain a regular supply. This is known as right time.

 (vi) *Right place:* Generally, the items are expected to deliver in the premise of the customers, is the right place.

 (vii) *Right mode of transportation:* The mode of transportation depends upon distance and time.

The right transportation is necessary for safety of materials during transportation.

(viii) *Right packaging:* The right packaging is necessary to prevent contamination of the product during transport and storage.

8 Write a note on "selection of supplier". (S. 96, 98, 01, 03, 05, 09; W. 99, 06)

☞ For selection of supplier, following points should be taken into consideration:

(i) For newcomer, the supplier may be manufacturer, distributor or wholesaler.

(ii) Proper selection of supplier ensures good quality and reasonable price and better services.

(iii) The information of various suppliers can be obtained from:

(a) Experienced owner

(b) Trade journals

(c) Indian pharmaceutical guide (IPG)

(d) Chamber of commerce.

(iv) The records and list of suppliers is to be prepared along with blacklisted supplier with reasons.

(v) New suppliers should be asked for the price, delivery and other terms and conditions.

(vi) The comparative statement of quotations should be prepared.

(vii) When the quality is standard the price should be compromised but there should not be any compromise on the quality.

(viii) The important points should be recorded regarding the suppliers are:

(i) Name, address, phone no., fax no., e-mail of supplier

(ii) Weekly holiday

(iii) Working hours

(iv) Names of representatives

(v) Names of companies with the suppliers

(vi) Names of products available

(vii) Terms and conditions like:

• Mode of payment

• Credit period

• Taxes

• Transportation charges

(viii) Blacklisted suppliers are separately recorded along with particular reasons.

(ix) Price of the products, etc.

9 Write a note on "credit information".

☞• The term credit is defined as a purchase without immediate cash payment.

• Sometimes, the total cost of purchase is very large and very difficult to carry liquid cash for purchase. Thus, due to above reason and to promote the trade, the suppliers offer credit facility.

• No credit is offered to the newcomers to avoid uncertainty.

• Sometimes, funds may not be available to the purchaser, it makes credit transaction as a compulsory part of the business.

• The purchaser is asked to make the payments within a specific duration of time, interest on payment may or may not be charged.

• Post-dated cheques are also accepted as credit facilities.

• Credit period:
   (a) For wholesalers—21 to 45 days.
   (b) For retailers—15 to 30 days.

Factors to be considered in offering credit:

(i) *Character:* Honesty, reputation and moral conduct.

(ii) *Capacity:* Knowledge, business experience, judgement, resourcefulness.

(iii) *Capital:* It includes liquid funds, assets, loans and long-term investments.

(iv) *Condition:* Internal and external factors offering a business.

10 Define "tender". Explain various types of tenders.

☞ Tender (S. 96, 97, 99, 03, 06, 07, 08; W. 98, 04, 05, 06)

A tender is the procedure of inviting prices of materials and terms and conditions of supply from the suppliers.

Types of Tenders

(a) *Oral tenders:* In this type, the suppliers are requested to visit the purchasing organisation and inform the prices of products. On receiving the information purchase orders are placed.

(b) *Single tender:* In this type, the purchase department appoints a person to enquire prices of the product in the market and to record the information.
- The supplier is selected who offers lowest price.
- This method is followed when the material is of little use.

(c) *Limited tender:* In this type, the tenders are invited from "approved suppliers" only.
- The purchaser has to make contact with suppliers. Generally, contact is done by written fashion. This method is used for purchasing proprietary products.

(d) *Open tender/public tender/advertise tender:*
- This method is followed when there are large number of suppliers and the requirement of materials is also large.
- In this type, purchaser gives advertisement in papers and trade journals. The suppliers are expected to prepare and deliver the price list or the quotations.
- The suppliers are also expected to send the price list in a sealed envelop and also send some small samples of the product.
- Sealed envelops are opened on a decided date and suitable supplier is selected. The order is placed to the supplier offering lowest prices.

11 Write a note on "contract". Define contract. Explain contract as purchase order. What points should be included in contract? (S. 96; W. 97, 02)

☞ **Contract**

"A contract is an agreement between two or more persons creating and defining obligations between two or more parties."
- Contract is considered as a purchase order. The purchase order represents the agreement between supplier and purchaser. Hence, purchase order is a contract.
- The following points should be covered during contract:

A. Draft

(i) Name and address of purchaser.

(ii) Name and address of supplier.

(iii) Purchase order no., reference no. and date.

(iv) Full description of items.

 (v) Quantity of each material.

 (vi) Rate and total amount of each material.

 (vii) Mode of transportation and date of delivery.

(viii) Packaging and forwarding charges, local taxes.

 (ix) Discount, if any.

 (x) After purchase services.

 (xi) Signature of the owner and the seal, stamp.

B. Legal Aspects

 (i) The purchase order should be legal and it should be accepted by the suppliers.

 (ii) The purchase order and the acceptance by the supplier should not be unlawful.

(iii) The person involved should have legal capacity to enter in contract.

(iv) Each party should give freedom to other party to fulfill promises and duties.

 (v) The objectives of the contract should be lawful.

12 What are various essential "elements of contract"?

☞ Elements of Contract

1. The offer should be legal.
2. There should be legal acceptance resulting in valid contract.
3. The agreement creates a legal relationship and if any party fails in fulfilling its role, the same is liable for punishment.
4. No unlawful method should be used in the offer and acceptance.
5. The parties in the agreement should have legal right to enter in the business.
6. Any minor or lunatic cannot enter in contract.
7. The object of activity should be lawful.
8. The agreement should not be impossible for performance.
9. The terms or words in the contract should be clear and should not mislead any party, otherwise it is not enforcible.

13 Define "price". What are various types of prices?

☞ Price

"The price refers to the amount of money at which a thing is valued."

Types of Prices

(i) *Firm price:* It is the price of material during contract period.

(ii) *Price in force:* It is the price at the time of despatch.

(iii) *Cost plus:* The supplier is allowed to have some % margin over the price.

(iv) *Guaranteed maximum price:* The purchaser asks the supplier to set maximum limit of cost.

(v) *Price adjustment:* Prices are settled by discussions.

14 What are the different methods of "pricing of materials"?

☞**A. FIFO (first in first out method) (W. 03):**

- The materials which are received first are issued first at the price at which they are purchased.
- Thus change in cost price, lot wise will not affect the sale.
- This method is used for the products with stable prices and less frequency of purchases and sale.

B. LIFO (last in first out method) (W. 03):

- In this method, the price of the latest product in the stock is used for calculating the value of issue material.
- It is used for the products, whose prices are changed very commonly.

C. Average cost method:

- Average price is calculated on the basis of the various prices of the materials.

$$\text{Average cost} = \frac{\text{Total value}}{\text{Number of items}}$$

D. Replacement price method:

- The prices are updated every day.
- The current prices are considered.

E. Inflated price method:

In this method, the wastage is added for the price calculation.

F. Standard pricing method:

It is the price fixed after careful observations of the competitors' activities, current expenditure and market trends.

15 How the retail price of formulation is calculated? (S. 06)

☞ Retail price of drug formulations is calculated as per DPCO as follows:

$$\text{Retail price} = [\text{MC} + \text{CC} + \text{PM} + \text{PC}] \times \left[1 + \frac{\text{MAPE}}{100}\right] + \text{ED}$$

Where,

RP	= Retail price
MC	= Material cost
CC	= Conversion cost
PM	= Cost of packaging material
PC	= Packaging cost
MAPE	= Maximum allowable postmanufacturing expenses
ED	= Excise duty.

16 Define "discount". Give types of discounts. (S. 04; W. 04)

☞ **Discount**

It is an offer either in cash or in terms of goods from manufacturer or wholesaler to retailer for stimulating the early payment.

Types of Discount

(a) *Trade discount:* It is given to either wholesaler or retailers for performing better marketing activities. A trade discount for a wholesaler normally ranges from 15 to 20%, for pharmacy 30 to 50%.

(b) *Quantity discount:* It is given when quantity of purchase is large. The discount ranges from 5 to 20%. Sometimes, discount is given in the form of free goods.

(c) *Cash discount:* Cash discount is smallest discount of all. A cash discount is given to a buyer for payment within a given period specified on the statement. It is normally 1 to 2% of total.

(d) *Serial discount:* In pharmacy, the series of discount is implied and typically will be 40% (trade discount), 10% (quantity discount) and 2% (cash discount). They are multiplied and subtracted in steps, beginning with the largest discount which is usually listed first.

▊17▊ Define codification of drugs. Give the advantages/ importance/objectives of codification. (S. 96, 97, 98, 00, 03, 04, 09; W. 96, 97, 98, 99, 01, 02)

☞ "Codification is the process of giving codes, symbols or numbers to a particular group of items for easy identification or classification of drugs."

Advantages/Objectives/Importance

   (i) For quick identification and short description of items (drugs).
  (ii) To codify each item on logical basis.
 (iii) To bring together various products having similar properties.
 (iv) It describes the drug briefly and thus saves time.
  (v) It helps in accounting process.
 (vi) It gives standardisation of variety of items.
(vii) It helps in computer feeding.

▊18▊ Describe various method of codification with their advantages and disadvantages. (S. 97, 98, 00, 05, 06, 08; W. 98, 01, 04, 06)

☞ **Methods of Codification**

   1. Alphabetical method
   2. Mnemonic method
   3. Numerical method
   4. Combined method

1. Alphabetical Method

In this method, English alphabets are assigned for dosage forms:
  For example: 'T' for tablets
                  'C' for capsules
                  'I' for injections

Advantages

  (i) Very simple method.
 (ii) Helps in defining location of product.
(iii) Brand names may be arranged alphabetically.

Disadvantages

(i) Dosage forms having similar alphabets cannot be coded by this method.

(ii) There is no flexibility in the system.

2. Mnemonic Method

In this method, active drugs are abbreviated with or without dosage forms.

For example: Diazepam tablet : DZP–T

     Diclofenac tablet : DPS–T

     Metronidazole tablet : MTZ–T

Advantages

(i) It is a simple method.

(ii) It is suitable when the number of items are few and the dosage forms are limited.

Disadvantages

(i) An abbreviation may have more than one full forms.

(ii) A register for decoding is essential.

(iii) It is not suitable for large number of products.

3. Numerical Method

It is the most simple method for traders and manufacturers in pharmacy.

In this method, numbers/digits are used as codes. It is divided into two:

(i) *Decimal method:* In this method, firstly number the pharmacological activity and then product.

For example: Antibiotics—1

     Penicillin-G : 1.1

     Streptomycin : 1.2

     Amoxicillin : 1.3

(ii) *Block method:* In this system, a set of numbers is reserved for a classified item.

For example: Tablets : 1 to 200

     Capsules : 201 to 300

     Creams : 301 to 400

Advantages

It has indefinite capacity, thus large number of drugs can be coded by this method.

4. Combined Method

It is a combination of alphabetical, mnemonic or numerical method.
For example: Respiratory system — RS

Ephedrine	:	RS–1
Salbutamol	:	RS–2
Theophylline	:	RS–3

Advantages

(i) Easy method.

(ii) Avoids confusion.

(iii) Avoids duplication of products and reduces inventory.

(iv) Reduces documentation in store department.

(v) Helps in computerisation of records.

Disadvantages

The systems of the body having same alphabets make confusions or cannot be coded.
For example: Respiratory system : RS

Reproductive system : RS

Inventory Control

1 Define inventory. Give importance of inventory.

☞ Inventory

Inventory is sum total of value of raw materials, semiprocessed goods, finished products, fuels, spare parts, at any given point of time.

Importance of Inventory

1. **Inventory is expenditure**
   - The inventory material has same value or cost in amount.
   - If excessive amount is locked in inventory, it will create problems in expenses like salaries of workers, light bills, etc.
   - If too less amount is employed in inventory, very little amount of money is available for processing, makes the business in danger.
   - Thus, to maintain inventory, right material should be made available to right worker at right time.

2. **Inventory increases profit**
   - Accurate purchase scheduling maintains adequate stock of materials.
   - By continuing the production and improving quality of products in minimum cost increases profitability.

2   What is inventory control? Give objectives of inventory control. (S. 96, 97, 98, 05, 07, 08, 09; W. 96, 97, 98, 00, 01, 04)

☞ **Inventory Control**

"Inventory control is an effective way to keep a watch over losses from misappropriation, damage, deterioration and carelessness and proper control over maintenance of stock."

Objectives of Inventory Control

1. To have a regular and uniform supply of materials.
2. To reduce or minimise investment in inventory.
3. To minimise wastage of raw material during storage.
4. To minimise misappropriation of materials.
5. To minimise thefts.
6. To obtain regular information about availability of product.
7. To maintain control over maintenance of stock.
8. To increase efficiency and smooth functioning of organisation.
9. To maintain proper utilisation of funds available.

3   Give the functions and importance of inventory control. (S. 02, 07, 08; W. 98, 99, 03, 05)

☞ 1. To keep the inventories as low as possible as per market conditions.
2. To remove "out of stock" or "excessive stock" conditions.
3. To maintain a sufficient stock of finished products to meet the market requirements.
4. To maintain proper records to estimate correct purchases.
5. To forecast the market and economic conditions of supply.
6. To take care of materials during storage period.
7. To provide a safety stock against strikes, transports, delays, etc.
8. To maintain proper leadtime during procurement of materials.

4   What are different methods, techniques and tools used in inventory control? (S. 97, 98, 01, 02, 03, 05; W. 97, 04)

☞ 1. ABC analysis
2. VED analysis

3. EOQ method
4. Setting of various levels
5. Perpetual inventory control system
6. Review of slow moving and fast moving items
7. Input-output ratio analysis
8. Want book
9. Effective purchase procedure.

5 Write a note on ABC analysis method of inventory control. (S. 02, 06, 09; W. 98, 01, 03, 06)

☞ ABC means Always Better Control system.

Definition

ABC analysis is a method of inventory control in which materials are divided into three categories as A-category, B-category and C-category, on the basis of cost and number of items.

A-category: Few items which are very costly.

B-category: The items which are moderately costly.

C-category: The large number of items which are very cheap.

According to international standards items are categorised as:

Category	% of items	% of investment/cost
A	08	75
B	25	20
C	67	05

Features of ABC Analysis

Nature	A-category items	B-category items	C-category items
1. Control	Very tight	Moderate	Loose
2. Level of management	Top level	Middle level	Low level
3. Safety stock	Nil	Low	Higher
4. Order frequency	High	Once in 3 months	Once in 6 months
5. Review period	1 month	3 months	6 months
6. Planning	Very accurate	Depending upon experience	Rough calculations

- *Advantages of ABC System of Inventory Control*
  1. It gives better control over costly items.
  2. It helps in developing scientific method of control.
  3. It helps in maintaining stock in a better way.
  4. It reduces storage cost.
  5. It maintains proper stock of ABC items.
  6. It enables better planning for purchase.
  7. It reduces clearical cost.

6 Define VED analysis. Describe in brief. Give importance. Write a note on VED analysis. (S. 96, 97, 99, 00, 01, 02, 03, 04, 06, 07; W. 96, 98, 01, 04)

☞ **VED Analysis**

Definition

VED analysis is a method of controlling and maintaining the stock of various types of materials of a specific group.

The word VED means:

V—Vital items

E—Essential items

D—Desirable items

This method is mainly used for spare parts. The spare parts are to be maintained to avoid disturbances in production process arising from machinary failure.

The spare parts are classified into 3 items:

1. **Vital items:** These are the items of which "out of stock" condition is never allowed. The unavailability will immediately stop the production process. Hence called vital items.

2. **Essential items:** These are the items of which "out of stock" condition is tolerated for few hours to one day, as the cost of unavailability is lesser than that of V items.

3. **Desirable items:** These are items having very less importance. So unavailability of items does not stop the production process. The out of stock condition can be tolerated up to one week.

Features of VED Analysis

	V-items	E-items	D-items
1.	Constant control and regular flow of material is necessary	Moderate control	Nil stock
2.	Moderate stock	Moderate stock	Low stock
3.	Out of stock condition not tolerated	Out of stock condition tolerated for few hours to 1 day	Out of stock condition is tolerated up to one week
4.	Items of great significance	Less significance	Negligible importance

7 What is EOQ? Give the methods of calculating EOQ. Mention advantages of EOQ or write a note on EOQ. (S. 96, 98, 99, 06, 07, 09; W. 96, 97, 98, 99, 00, 01, 02, 03, 04)

☞ **EOQ**

It is the balance between "ordering cost" and "inventory carrying cost".

"It is the number of units per order to be purchased which will minimise both inventory carrying cost and ordering cost."

The correct quantity to buy is the quantity at which ordering cost and inventory carrying cost will be minimum.

There are two major components of EOQ:

(a) Inventory carrying cost (S. 96, 97, 99; W. 99, 02)

It includes:

(i) Rent/cost of storage

(ii) Storage facilities provided

(iii) Cost of handling materials

(iv) Special facilities like refrigerator, air conditioning

(v) Amount of interest payable

(vi) Salary of store keeper and other staff.

(b) Ordering cost: It is the cost of placing order.

(i) Cost of stationary

(ii) Cost of postage, telephone, fax, e-mail, etc.

Methods of Calculating EOQ

(a) Formula method:

$$EOQ = \sqrt{\frac{2UO}{IC}}$$

U = Use of material per year
O = Ordering cost
C = Cost of one unit
I = Inventory carrying cost.

(b) Graphical method:

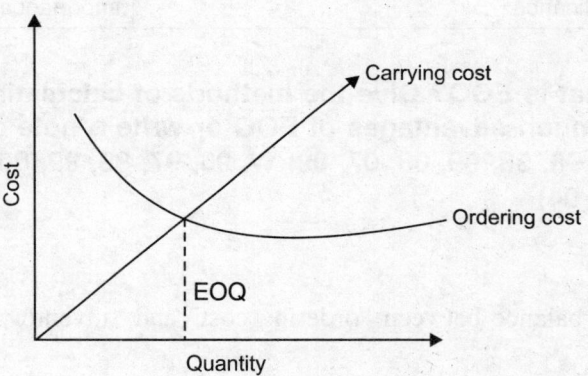

(c) Tabulation method: Figures are written in a separate column.

Advantages of EOQ

1. Simple method
2. Widely used
3. Number of orders to be placed in a given period of time can be calculated
4. Purchase schedule can be prepared
5. Maintains minimum inventory.

8 Write a note on various stock levels. Give the importance/objective of setting various stock levels.

☞ **Objectives of Setting Various Stock Levels**

1. To maintain uniform flow of materials in the business.
2. To supply the materials uniformly to production department.

3. To minimise the investment in materials.
4. To achieve uniformity in quality and quantity of finished products.

Important Stock Levels in Inventory Control

(a) **Maximum stock level (S. 96, 99, 04, 05; W. 99, 98, 01, 05, 06):** It is the upper limit of stock beyond which the stock of any item should not be allowed to increase.

Maximum stock level = Reordering level + Reorder quantity – (Minimum consumption) × (Minimum lead time)

(b) **Minimum stock level (S. 96, 98, 04, 05; W. 96, 97, 01, 05, 06):** It is the lower limit of stock below which the stock of any item should not be allowed to fall.

Minimum stock level = Reordering level – (Normal consumption × Normal lead time)

(c) **Reorder level (S. 96, 99, 05; W. 98, 99, 01, 05):** It is the level of stock of any item at which next purchase procedure is started. It is the level in between maximum and minimum stock levels.

Reorder level = Maximum lead time × Maximum consumption rate

(d) **Safety stock (S. 96, 97, 98, 99, 00, 08, 09; W. 98, 01, 02):** The quantities of stock below the minimum stock levels are considered as safety stocks.
They are utilised in emergency periods like strikes.

(e) **Danger level (W. 05):** When the quantity of stock falls below safety stock or minimum level it is known as danger level.

---

9 **How will you detect the slow and nonmoving items in a drug store? OR What steps are taken to detect slow and nonmoving items in the drug store? OR Write a note on review on slow and nonmoving item in inventory control. (W. 03)**

☞ This technique is useful for small scale traders as well as for manufacturer.

The principle of this method is every material should be consumed at the earliest, it releases the investment and increases cost effectiveness of business.

Steps taken to detect slow and nonmoving items in the drug store

   (a) Periodic report: A monthly or periodic report on the stock of nonmoving item is prepared which indicates regarding its purchase, consumption and balance in hand.

   (b) Obsolete items:
- These are the items which become useless due to change in design, cost, etc.
- Such slow and nonmoving, obsolete items should be detected and should be utilised and further purchase should be totally stopped.

   (c) Moving ratios:
- Moving ratio shows the turnover of items and slow moving items and nonmoving items can be calculated.
- Slow moving items are those which require more time for consumption.

10 **What do you mean by "input-output ratio analysis"? Give advantages.**

☞ **Definition**

Input-output ratio is a ratio between quantity of material charged to the production process and the quantity of material in the final output.

$$\text{Input-output ratio} = \frac{\text{Quantity of material used for production}}{\text{Quantity of final product}}$$

Advantages

1. It shows efficiency of the manufacturing department.
2. It indicates suitability of raw materials.
3. It gives the total cost of raw materials in finished goods.

11 **Write a note on "perpetual inventory control" system. (S. 05, 06; W. 04, 05)**

☞ **Perpetual Inventory Control System**

Perpetual inventory control is the spontaneous process of checking and recording of the stock, in which receipt, issue and balance of material is done regularly.

The perpetual method consists of:
1. Store keepers ledger
2. Bin card method
3. Continuous stock taking

1. Store keepers ledger
- Ledger is the register in which one or more pages are kept for single item.
- The ledger is to be maintained by store keeper.
- The balance of stocks is calculated 4–5 days before the order date.

2. Bin card method
- The bin cards are the information cards for each item.
- The bin cards provide the information at a glance.
- These are somewhat thick and used to record the receipts and issued entries.
- The bin cards are numbered serially and arranged in a filling cabinet or special drawer.

3. Continuous stock taking
- Some persons are appointed by management for this special duty (inspectors).
- The inspectors cross check the entries in store ledger and bin card. They also verify the stocks physically.
- Any variation in the stock is immediately informed to higher management.

Advantages of Perpetual System

(i) Overstocking and understocking are avoided.

(ii) Without disturbing routine, records can be checked.

(iii) It provides physical verification of stocks.

(iv) Any clerical mistake can be pointed out.

(v) Timely actions can be taken in cases of shortage.

(vi) The balance in stock can be known at any time.

12 **Explain "effective purchase procedure" as a method of inventory control. (S. 06; W. 05)**

☞ **Effective Purchase Procedure**

The effective purchase procedure involves three main activities.
1. Following the purchase schedule.

2. Taking decisions at correct times.
3. Studying market conditions, government policies and adjusting consumption of products continuously.

The steps to be taken during effective purchase are:

(i) Feeling need of material.
(ii) Checking stocks available.
(iii) Asking for price lists/quotations/tenders.
(iv) Selection of suppliers.
(v) Negotiations with suppliers.
(vi) Forwarding purchase order.
(vii) Making provisions of the finance required.
(viii) Receiving the material.
(ix) Quality analysis of material.
(x) Physical verification of received materials.
(xi) Checking the accuracy of bills.
(xii) Making payments.
(xiii) Recording the materials in registers.

Advantages

(a) It acts as a guide for further action
(b) It provides accuracy and pleasure of purchasing.
(c) The documents are prepared for legal safety.
(d) In certain business, purchase mannuals are prepared.

13 **What is scrap? Explain types of scrap. How can scrap be disposed of (controlled)? (S. 97, 03, 06, 08, 09; W. 98, 06)**

☞ Scrap

"Scrap is an occasional residue obtained from various manufacturing processes."

Examples of Scraps

(a) Spoiled raw materials
(b) Rejected components
(c) Defective materials
(d) Nonusable parts and equipments
(e) Waste from production department
(f) Nonusable packing materials.

Classification/Types of Scrap

1. **Legitimate scrap:** The scrap which can be predetermined in advance due to manufacturing operations, e.g. granules or powders remaining after manufacturing process.
2. **Administrative scrap:** It is the scrap material arising from changed policies of administration about formulation, packaging, labelling, etc.
3. **Defective scrap:** This scrap results from substandard raw materials and poor skill in workers handling such materials and equipments.

Control of Scrap

1. Careful designing of products.
2. Use of good quality raw materials and equipments.
3. Skilled workers should be appointed.
4. Using standard operating procedures.

Disposal of Scrap

1. It can be sold to other organisations at cheaper prices.
2. It can be recycled into useful materials for subsequent production of basic products.
3. Grade the materials, it gives good return in terms of money.
4. Tenders are invited if quantity of scrap is large.
5. Advantage of scrap disposal is that it releases the space.

14 **What do you mean by "surplus" items? Give its causes. How can surplus items be disposed of? (S. 96, 97, 01, 02, 08, 09; W. 97, 98, 01, 06)**

☞ **Surplus**

"The surplus items are those which are the excess items than reasonable requirements."

Examples:

(i) Rejected components
(ii) Defective parts
(iii) Expiry items
(iv) Dead stock items

Causes of Surplus

1. Surplus may also arise due to fall in sale of particular product.
2. Surplus may arise due to some problems in production.
3. Surplus may arise due to unwanted purchase mistake.
4. Surplus may arise due to purchasing in bulk due to lower prices of materials.

Disposal of Surplus

1. Surplus should be disposed of by returning the material to the supplier by replacing it with the other required material.
2. Surplus can also be disposed of by calling tender if the quantity is very large.
3. Surplus can also be disposed of by negotiation to other consumers of same items.
4. If possible, surplus can be reprocessed into useful raw materials for subsequent production of basic products.
5. Disposal of surplus releases space.

15 Write a note on "lead time". (S. 97, 98, 01, 02; W. 96, 98, 01, 02, 03, 06)

☞ **Lead time**

"The time required from placement of an order to the time it is received and approved by quality control department."

The lead time has two components:

(a) **Administrative lead time:** It includes the time taken by organisation to complete the purchase procedure calling price lists, analysis of price list, making enquiries and negotiations, etc.

(b) **Suppliers lead time:**
 • It includes time required for communication and transportation of materials.
 • It includes collection, packaging of order, transportation.
 • If delivery is by post, then postal delays may increase lead time.

Sales Promotion

1 **Define sales promotion. Describe various techniques/ modes/tools/methods used in sales promotion. (S. 01, 02, 09; W. 01, 03, 04, 05)**

☞ **Sales Promotion**

The technique or method used to improve or promote the sale of products is known as sale promotion.

Techniques of Sales Promotion

(a) **Free samples:** Many manufacturers use this method to introduce a new product into the market. The products in small packages are distributed free.

(b) **Trading coupons:** They are issued to the customers through retailers in proportion of size of purchase. Minimum number of coupons are to be collected and sent to the manufacturer. A product in free is given against the collection of coupons.

(c) **Coupons:** A coupon is a certificate that declares some discount to the holder. They are distributed through mail, newspapers or retailers. The retailers are allowed to handover the products to coupon holders. The difference in payment is adjusted by manufacturer.

(d) **Premium or bonus offer:** This method gives certain quantity of product free of cost or it may be:

(i) **With pack premium:** A gift is inserted along with container, e.g. spoon with baby food.

(ii) Reusable container.

(iii) **Free in the mail premium:** A free gift is offered to the customer on sending proof of purchase.

(e) **Price contests:** It is a very common and famous technique. The contests are published in newspapers or magazines and winners receive an attractive package of gift.

(f) **Fairs and exhibitions:** They are organised to display and popularise the product. One or more manufacturers unite together and arrange such exhibitions.

2 Define the term 'market'. Classify market. (S. 07)

☞ **Market**

Market is the geographical area where seller and customer come in contact.

Classification of Market

Market can be classified in various ways:

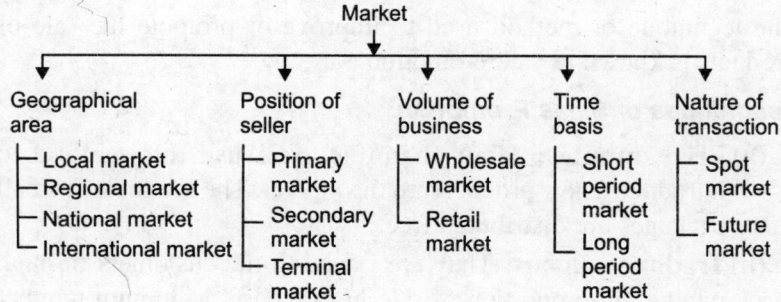

3 Define "marketing". Explain functions of marketing. (W. 03)

☞ **Marketing**

"Marketing means the performance of business activities that direct the flow of goods and services from producers to consumers."

Functions of Marketing

1. **Buying:** Buying is the starting function of marketing.

2. **Assembling:** It is a collection of same or variety of products from different places.

3. **Selling:** It means to sell the goods and services and to earn profit.

4. **Advertisement:** Advertisement makes potential buyers aware of new products available in the market.

5. **Transportation:** Transportation creates a place utility. Goods can reach the places where they are in demand.

6. **Storage and warehousing:** The goods should be stored till the demand is received. Warehouse is a place where goods are stored, preserved, protected against risk of theft, contamination, fire, etc.

7. **Financing:** Finance is the lubricant of marketing machinery.

8. **Risk bearing:** Marketing process has a risk of many kinds at every stage, such as accidents, fire, theft, earthquake, flood, change in demand, change in price.

9. **Market information:** It means all the facts, opinions and other information used in marketing of goods.

10. **Standardisation:** Means to check the standards of drugs such as colour, size, quality, purity, etc. to assure the customers about the quality.

11. **Grading:** Means classification of goods into different classes on the basis of size and quality.

12. **Branding:** To identify groups of seller and to differentiate the products from various competitors.

13. **Packing and packaging:** Packing means the wrapping and placing of goods in suitable container.

Packaging means putting the goods in packages, e.g. bags, boxes, cans, etc.

4 Define market research. What are the objectives and advantages of market research? (S. 96, 97, 02, 05, 08, 09; W. 99, 06)

☞ **Market Research**

"It is the process of gathering, recording and analysis of market data to identify present and potential customers."

Objectives

(i) To identify present and future customers.

(ii) To increase the demand of product.

(iii) To judge the customer's preferences about packaging, size, price and design, etc.

(iv) To find out new markets for existing products.

(v) To take the feedback of products from market.

Advantages of Market Research (S. 09; W. 01, 03)

(i) To introduce new products in the market.

(ii) Source of information about customer's response to any product.

(iii) Competitor's activities can be observed.

(iv) Gives an idea regarding future trends in market.

(v) Discovery of new markets while maintaining present markets.

(vi) To earn more profits by modifying price structure, packaging or design.

(vii) To study government policies.

(viii) To bring forward a solution to any other problem.

(ix) To develop new product.

(x) Advantage for new line of product.

(xi) To maintain a planned production.

(xii) To increase effectiveness of existing channels of distribution.

5 **How is market research done? Explain the procedure of market research. What are various steps involved in market research? (W. 96, 97)**

☞ **Procedure/Steps involved in Market Resarch**

(a) **To fix the problem:** It is most basic step and it makes the research focus.

(b) **Determination of specific objectives:** It involves goals and aims of research.

(c) **Determination of geographical area** in which research is carried out.

(d) **Selection of agency or representatives:** Manufacturer may appoint external agency for the job when scope of research is large.

(e) **Collection of information:** The agency works in a given area and collects the information from various sources:

(i) *Internal source*: It means information is collected from the organisation/manufacturer.

(ii) *External source*:

   I. **Primary information data** from salesman, dealers and customers.

   II. **Secondary information data** from newspapers, trade magazines, journals and government publications, etc.

(f) **Analysis of information:** The information collected from every source is brought together and analysed.

(g) **Drawing conclusions:** A summary of report of analysis and highlights of data collected are enlisted.

(h) **Preparation of report:** A report is a statement of facts and suggestive actions to be taken to impliment answers to the problems.

(i) **Making recommendations:** The conclusions drawn are reported to the manufacturer.

In this way market research is complete.

6 What are different sources of market research? (S. 08)

☞ Market research involves the collection and analysis of information. There are two types of sources:

(a) **Internal source:** The information is collected from persons working inside the organisation, i.e. sales turnover, expenditure, advertisement expenditure and transport, etc.

(b) **External source:** The information is collected from persons working outside the organisation.

The external sources may be:

   (i) *Primary sources*: The information is collected from:
   - Salesmen   - Retailers
   - Dealers   - Distributors
   - Consumers.

   (ii) *Secondary sources*: The information is taken from:
   - Trade press
   - Published survey reports
   - Trade associations
   - Government and internal publications.

7 **What are different survey methods of market research? OR What are different methods of collecting information (data) in market research? (S. 98, 03, 06; W. 99, 05)**

☞ **(a) Personal interview method:** It involves collection of information by asking questions. It involves face to face communication between reseacher and responder.

(b) Mail/postal survey method: It this method some questions are posted to the responder and he is asked to answer within given time.

(c) Telephone survey method: Information is collected by asking questions on telephone.

(d) Panel method: In this method, a group of persons is selected to collect the information about the product. The persons may be wholesaler, retailer or consumer. The necessary conclusions can be drawn from observations made by panel.

(e) Observation method: In this method, no any question is asked, only the activities of traders and consumers are observed.

(f) Experimentation method:
- It is a common method in marketing.
- Before introducing new product in the market, manufacturer distributes samples of products.
- After use of products, manufacturer collects opinions of consumers about quality, packaging or prices of product.

8 **What is salesmanship? What are the duties and responsibilities of 'salesman'? (S. 96, 97, 99, 02; W. 99, 00, 01)**

☞ **Salesmanship**

"Salesmanship is an art of convincing the people to buy the product of the business, offering them purchase satisfaction."

Duties and Responsibilities of Salesman

1. To promote sales of company products.
2. To provide information regarding products to the physician and remind him old products.
3. To build a better image of company in eyes of physician.
4. To maintain an adequate distribution of products in the market.

5. To provide feedback information from the physician, chemist and wholesalers.
6. To maintain a close contact with outlet channels to have smooth distribution.
7. To provide free samples to physicians for trials on patients.
8. To adjust the expiry goods and breakage available with retailer or wholesaler.
9. To cooperate in market research.

9 **What are different qualities of a 'salesman'? OR Enlist different qualities of a salesman should possess. OR What qualities of a person should possess to become a successful salesman? (S. 97, 99, 00, 03, 05, 06, 08, 09; W. 96, 97, 99, 00, 01, 02, 06)**

☞ **Qualities of Salesman**

(a) Physical qualities (personal qualities)
(i) Sound health
(ii) Smiling face
(iii) Clear voice
(iv) Natural tone
(v) Pleasing personality
(vi) Should be well dressed and cheerful appearance
(vii) Hardworking and ability to impress the customers.

(b) Mental qualities:
(i) Sound memory
(ii) Good imagination
(iii) Balanced thinking and foresight
(iv) Positive thinking, open-minded
(v) Emotionally balanced, presence of mind.

(c) Social qualities:
(i) Liking to mix with others
(ii) Good conversional ability
(iii) Sound character
(iv) Honest and cooperative
(v) Sincere and polite
(vi) Good listener
(vii) Good patience.

(d) Vocational qualities:
  (i) Should have technical knowledge of product
  (ii) Knowledge about business activities
  (iii) Should have minimum academic qualification
  (iv) Should know the composition of market
  (v) Should know about government policies and marketing policies of competitors.

10 **What are various steps involved in the selling process? OR Describe the sale procedure or selling procedure.**

☞ The process of selling consists of following steps:

(a) **Presale preparation:** In this step, salesmen are appointed. They are trained and motivated to make sale. They are trained in reference with product information, communication skill, codified products, handling and others.

(b) **Prospecting:** The salesman should identify the needs of customers.

(c) **Approaching:** It includes salesman introduction on customers welcome. The salesman should explain qualities of product. He should assure good service to the customer.

(d) **Presentation:** The product should be shown to the customer. The salesman tries to convince the customer about satisfaction of needs. He explains technical details of the product.

(e) **Dealing with objections:** It is a right of customers to ask the queries. Generally the questions asked should be regarding quality, quantity and price of the product. Salesman should be very cool, quiet and patient, while dealing with objections.

(f) **Providing additional information:** The complete information about working instructions, safety measures should be provided to the customers.

(g) **Closing the sales:** After showing the product and discussion some time is given to the customer for his thinking and right decision. If customer satisfies with product then products are handed over to customer and money is received.

(h) **Additional sales as per requirement of customer:** If customer satisfies with the product, he will give an additional order as per requirements.

(i) **Follow up (after sales service):** It includes after sale services and maintenance of records of customers. It also creates a permanent relationship with the customers.

11 What are the features of salesmanship? Give importance or significance of salesmanship.

☞ **Features of Salesmanship**

1. It is an art of selling.
2. It consists of influencing one mind by others.
3. Salesmanship is related with winning regular customers.
4. Due to salesmanship seller and buyer both are benefited.
5. Providing knowledge to the customer is essential part of salesmanship.

Importance or Significance of Salesmanship

1. It increases sales of the business and profits.
2. It is an instrument of creating permanent demand for certain products.
3. It is useful in improving living standard of customers.
4. It creates job opportunities to young and energetic people.

12 Define advertisement. Give objectives and functions of advertisement.

☞ **Advertisement**

Advertisement is an art used to familiarise the public with product by informing its description, use, price, and its superiority over other brands, etc.

Objectives of Advertisement (S. 00)

1. To create a demand for new products.
2. To maintain the existing demand of the product.
3. To enlarge market of the product.
4. To increase sales.
5. To help the salesman.
6. To educate the people about application and use of product.
7. To improve goodwill of the manufacturer.

8. To help the manufacturer in facing competition.
9. To warn the customers about imitation.
10. To reduce number of salesman and to establish direct link between producers and customers.

Functions/Significance/Importance of Advertisement (S. 04, 09)

1. It encourages prospective buyers to purchase the product.
2. It educates the people about the product or service.
3. It reduces number and responsibility of salesman.
4. It reduces seasonal fluctuations in the demand of the product.
5. It creates job opportunities.
6. It helps to introduce new products in the market.
7. It may remove the middleman.
8. It increases the goodwill of organisation.
9. It helps in increasing growth of the organisation.
10. It is a tool of sale promotion.

13 What is advertising? What are different medias of advertisement? (S. 99, 02, 06; W. 96, 97, 99)

☞ **Advertising**

"Advertising is defined as the sum total of all the activities involved in presenting to a group, a nonpersonal, oral or visual, openly sponsered message regarding a product, service or idea."

Medias for Advertising

(a) **Print media/press advertising:**
   It consists of:
   (i) *Newspapers*: It may be local, regional or national news-papers.
   (ii) *Magazines*: They may be weekly, monthly, biweekly periodicals.
   (iii) *Trade journals*: Advertisements in trade journals are more informative.
   (iv) *Pamplets*: These are colourful and distributed personally or randomly.
(b) **Audio-advertising:** Radios, sound systems.

(c) *Audiovisual media*:
 (i) *Television*: It is very popular and effective medium and very costly. Local area network, regional area network, national network can be selected.
 (ii) *Film presentations*:
  I. Audiovisual cassettes
  II. CDs or documentaries

(d) *Outdoor advertisement*: Posters, cards, banners, wall writing, road painting, electronic, neo-signs.

(e) *Mail advertising*: To physicians, retailers or customers.

(f) *Personal contact*: Sales representatives, medical representatives.

(g) *Displays*: Window displays, fairs and exhibitions.

14 Give advantages and disadvantages of advertisement. (S. 01, 02)

☞ *Advantages of Advertisement*

1. It helps to introduce new product in the market.
2. It increases prospective buyers to purchase products.
3. It helps to expand the market.
4. It increases sale.
5. It helps to overcome competition.
6. It educates the people about product and service.
7. It assists the salesman.
8. It develops relationship/communication between manufacturer and customer.
9. It creates job opportunities.
10. It is a source of income to newspapers, television channels, etc.
11. It increases goodwill of the manufacturer.
12. It may remove the middleman.
13. It keeps the demand of product constant.
14. It helps in increasing the growth of company.

Disadvantages of Advertisement

1. It increases cost of the product.
2. Sometimes, it creates an artificial demand of the product.
3. It leads to monopoly of the product.
4. Some advertisements may mislead the society.

5. Sometimes meaning of words, photographs, scenes may be harmful to morality of the society.
6. A large amount is invested before sale of the product.

15 **Write a note on "window display". (S. 96, 97, 99, 05, 06, 09; W. 96, 99, 00, 04, 06)**

☞ **Window Display**

"Window display is most effective and direct method of attracting customers and is one of the ways of advertising."

– Window display is commonly done through retailers.
– Window displays attract the customers into shop and make their mind to buy certain goods which are displayed.
– Small window display is called "shadowbox" and displays are usually 1 to 1.25 meter and located at sides of stores.

Objectives

1. To attract the likely customers about newly introduced products.
2. To inform customer about varieties of products available.
3. To assist the salesman.
4. To increase the sale of OTC products.
5. To make good impression.

Location of Window Display

1. On both sides of entrance of drug store.
2. Public places like railway stations, bus stands, restaurants, hotels, motels, etc. (for luxurious items).

Products Displayed

Home remedies, cosmetics, oral liquids, toilet preparation in attractive packages.

Essentials of Window Display

1. Display should not be crowdy.
2. Products should be changed periodically or seasonwise.
3. Display should be attractive and effective.
4. Sufficient space between the products displayed.
5. Products displayed should be free from dust.

Presentation

1. Back drops, steps, carpets, illumination system with colour combinations may attaract the customers.
2. Generally red colour catches the sight very easily while green colour is given least importance.

Advantages

1. Sale promotion
2. Media of advertising
3. To maintain name of brand all over
4. To increase goodwill of company.

Recruitment, Training, Evaluation and Compensation of Pharmacist

1 Define recruitment. What are various sources of recruitment?

☞ **Recruitment**

"Recruitment is the process of selecting appropriate persons for the specified job in the organisation."

Sources of Recruitment

There are two sources of searching suitable candidates for the job.
(a) External source
(b) Internal source.

(a) External source

In this case, the candidates are invited in the organisation from open society. Applications are invited and suitable candidates are selected. The empolyer may obtain the information from educational institution or employment exchange.

Advantages

(i) Availability of suitable persons and wide chance in selection.
(ii) It brings fresh blood and fresh ideas in the organisation.

Disadvantages

(i) Demoralisation of existing employees.
(ii) The existing employee may not cooperate the new employee.

(b) Internal source

The employee is selected from the existing employees only. Promotions, demotions or transfers are the ways of filling the vacancy by using internal source.

Advantages

   (i) More suitable in large scale organisation.
  (ii) Improves moral of existing employees.
 (iii) It promotes loyality.
 (iv) Requires less training to employee.
  (v) It is economical.

Disadvantages

   (i) Internal sources are finite and capable persons may not be available.
  (ii) Qualified person may not be available.
 (iii) Lack of new ideas and concepts.
 (iv) Less tendency of hardworking.

2 **How will you recruit pharmacist? OR Exlpain procedure/process of recruitment. (S. 00, 01, 02, 05, 06; W. 96, 97, 98, 99)**

☞ The steps involved in recruitment are:

   (a) Identifying the job for which person is to be appointed.
   (b) **Advertisement:** Advertisements are published in newspapers about the nature of job and expectations from candidates. The candidates are asked to submit biodata.
   (c) **Collection of applications:** All the applications received are collected and registered.
   (d) **Scrutiny of applications:** Incomplete applications are rejected. The candidates satisfying minimum expectations are also rejected.
   (e) **Tests:** The applicants are invited for testing their knowledge and intellect. Test papers consist of objective questions which are based on general knowledge, vocational, logic, etc.
   (f) **Primary interview:** The suitable candidates from the report of above test are invited for primary interview. It involves questioning on knowledge, family background, personality, ambitions, working ability.

(g) **Reference check:** The history of candidate is checked from local police station and enquiries are carried out.

(h) **Final interview:** It involves discussion with candidates about job, geographical area, technical details about organisation, salaries expected, etc.

(i) **Physical examination/medical checkup:** After selection, candidate should submit fitness certificate.

(j) **Issuing appointment order:** Appointment orders are given to selected candidates.

(k) **Receiving joining letters:** After joining, the candidates should submit joining letter to the higher authority.

3 What do you mean by training to pharmacist? OR Define training. Give need and importance. Enlist types of training. (S. 97, 02, 05, 08, 09; W. 99)

☞ **Training**

"Training is an organised process to increase knowledge and skill of the candidate for a specific job."

Need and Importance of Training

(i) To increase productivity of candidate.

(ii) To reduce supervision required.

(iii) For minimum wastage of material.

(iv) To prevent accidents.

(v) To increase the efficiency.

(vi) To increase moral of candidate.

(vii) For other developments of the candidates.

Points to be Covered during Training (W. 03)

(i) Organisation framework.

(ii) Daily routine and special duties.

(iii) Rules, conventions, norms and policies of the organisation.

(iv) Study of course material and literature.

(v) Method of dealing with objections of customers.

(vi) Communication skills.

(vii) Technical knowledge.

Methods/Types of Training

(a) **Job training:** To improve vocational and professional skills of the candidates.
(b) **Craft training:** To improve personal skills of the candidate.
(c) **Induction training:** To introduce new concepts or modern methods.
(d) **Training for promotion.**
(e) **Refresher training:** To revise vocational knowledge of the candidate.

4 **What do you mean by evaluation of pharmacist? How is evaluation of pharmacist done? (S. 97, 99, 04, 05, 09; W. 98, 00, 06)**

☞ **Evaluation**

"Evaluation is a systematic process for measuring performance of candidate in terms of job requirement, need and importance."

Need of Evaluation

(i) For comparison in workers.
(ii) Improvements in working in workers.
(iii) Discussion about promotion, demotion, lay off.
(iv) It develops confidence in workers.
(v) It is psychological pressure on the workers.

Method of Evaluation

Evaluation of candidates is done by using following sheet.

Evaluation sheet	
Name of the organisation	:
Address of organisation	:
Evaluation period	: from .... to ....
Name of candidate	:
Date of joining	:
Past experience	:

Criteria assessed	Remarks
(i) Appearance	XXX
(ii) Personality	XXX
(iii) Alertness	XXX
(iv) Courtesy and attitude	XXX
(v) Cooperation with other workers	XXX
(vi) Product knowledge	XXX
(vii) Communication capacity	XXX
(viii) Selling capacity	XXX
(ix) Suggestive selling	XXX
(x) Self-improvement	XXX
Total	**XXXX**

Evaluation is carried out after specific period. Either marks or grades are given for each criterion and total is done. Summary record of each candidate is prepared. Candidates with higher marks show great performance.

5 What do you mean by compensation? Give methods of compensation. (S. 08; W. 99, 05, 06)

☞ **Compensation**

"The compensation is the payment made to the candidate for his services to the organisation."

It is also known as remuneration to a worker.

Purpose/Need of Compensation

(i) To retain good employees.

(ii) It encourages them to work hard.

(iii) It maintains good and smooth working of organisation.

The compensation/remuneration should be:

(i) Attractive

(ii) Flexible (should change from time to time)

(iii) Should be uniform

(iv) Simple in nature

(v) Includes promotions, bonus, gifts and incentives.

Types of Compensation

(a) **Salary method:** It is a popular method. Salaries are paid every week or every month.

Advantages:

(i) Simple and economical

(ii) Provides safety to the candidates

(iii) Gives job satisfaction.

(b) **Commission method:** It is popular in marketing field. It is performance-oriented.

Advantages:

(i) Promotes hard working

(ii) Promotes efficiency

(iii) Helps in identifying active and inactive workers.

Disadvantages:

(i) Does not give security.

(ii) Does not offer job satisfaction.

(iii) Applies psychological pressure (stress) in the workers in uncertain market conditions.

(c) **Pooled commission method:** The amount of commission is distributed equally in all agents. The method is not popular in the workers.

(d) **Combined salary and commission method:** The commission is given on extra work done by candidate. The salaries are also given for regular job.

Banking and Finance

1 Define bank. What are different kinds/types of banks? (S. 97, 99, 01, 02, 07, 09; W. 97, 02, 05)

☞ **Bank**

"Bank is an institution which undertakes purchase and sale of money."
"Bank is an institution which deals in money and providing credit."
"Bank is a place of transaction of money."

Kinds/Types of Bank

(a) **Saving banks:** A person deposits his surplus money in the saving bank and receives some interest on it.
It cultivates habit of saving money in society.

(b) **Commercial banks:** It accepts money from depositors and makes the loans advances. They operate in the difference between rate of interest on loans or deposits.

(c) **Mixed banks:** They undertake the function of commercial bank and saving bank.

(d) **Cooperative banks:** They are formed on cooperative principles. They are supported by state or central governments.
Cooperative banks can be classified:
   (i) Primary credit society
   (ii) District central bank
   (iii) State cooperative bank.

(e) **Land development banks:**
   • The ownership is of state government.

- The finance required by them is partly satisfied by state and partly by central government.
- These are located at district places and provide loans to agriculture sector with minimum interest.

(f) **Industrial banks:**
- These banks work for industrial sector.
- They may be financed by governemnt or private sector.
- They provide long-term or medium-term loans to industries with higher rate of interest.

(g) **Export-import banks:** They assist exporters and importers. They are financed by governemnt and others. They provide short-term loans with highest rate of interest.

2 Explain various functions of bank. (S. 97, 99, 01, 02, 05, 07, 08, 09; W. 97, 02, 06)

☞ The functions of bank are of two types:
1. Primary functions
2. Secondary functions.

1. Primary Functions

(a) **Accepting deposits:** A bank accepts deposits in various ways. The ways of deposition are as follows:
   (i) Saving account deposits
   (ii) Cumulative account deposits
   (iii) Fixed deposits
   (iv) Cash certificates
   (v) Current account deposits

(b) **Making loan advances:** A bank provides loans to individual person or organisation.
Types of loans:
   (i) General loan
   (ii) Cash credit
   (iii) Overdraft
   (iv) Purchases and discounting bills.

2. Secondary Functions

(a) **Utility functions:**
   (i) Safe custody, e.g. lockers

  (ii) Travellers cheque and gift cheques

  (iii) Dealing with foreign exchange

  (iv) Help in capital issues

  (v) Providing trade information

  (vi) Advise on financial matters.

 (b) **Agency functions**

  (i) Collection of cheques, bills, and interest, commission

  (ii) Accepting insurance premium and instalments

  (iii) Sales and purchase of securities

  (iv) Transfer of funds

  (v) Functions as a trustee.

3   Define cheque, drawer, drawee. Mention different kinds/types of cheques. (S. 97, 02, 04, 07; W. 98, 99)

☞ **Cheque:** A cheque is an order given by drawer to the bank to issue amount of money mentioned therein to the drawee.

Drawer: Drawer writes the cheque and issues it to drawee.

Drawee: Drawee receives cheque from drawer and presents it in bank.

Bank: Bank issues money to drawee by taking it away from drawer's account.

Kinds/Types of Cheque

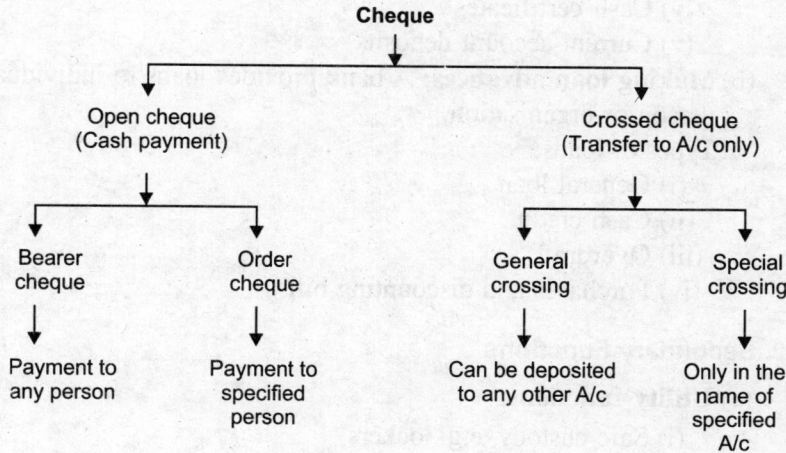

4 Give the advantages of cheque.

☞ **Advantages of Cheque**

1. Cheque is the helpful instrument which avoids risk in carrying cash.
2. Crossed cheques ensure safety in payments.
3. Endorsement is possible.
4. The counter foil serves record purpose.
5. On back side of counter foil, signature of receiver of cheque can be taken which is a proof.
6. The counter foils can be submitted in court of law as proof.

5 Define finance. Give functions/purpose/uses of finance. (S. 97, 98, 02, 04, 05, 06; W. 96, 98, 99, 00)

☞ **Finance**

Finance is a provision of money at the time when business requires it.

Functions of Finance

1. To acquire land, building, machinery and equipment.
2. To purchase raw material and other necessary items.
3. To pay salaries and wages.
4. To maintain regular supply of product in the market.
5. To pay rent insurance, taxes and advertising expenses.
6. To allow credits to wholesalers.

6 What are different sources of finance? Enlist important sources of finance. (S. 97, 99, 02, 04, 05, 06, 09; W. 96, 97, 98, 99, 00, 01, 06)

☞

Sources of finance		
Long-term source (for more than 5 years)	**Medium-term source (for 1–5 years)**	**Short-term source (for less than 1 year)**
• Equity shares • Debentures • Public deposits • Loans from financial institutions • Ploughing back of earning	• Preference shares • Medium-term loans • Debentures • Public deposits • Bank loans • Loans from financial institutes	• Cash credit • Overdraft • Trade credit • Advances from customers • Installment credit • Recirculation of profit

7 Define the terms "share" and "debenture".

☞ **a. Share**

When the capital is divided into smaller units, each unit is described as share.

There are two types of shares:
1. Preference shares
2. Equity shares.

b. Debenture

Debenture is a document under company seal which provides for the payment of principal sum and interest thereon at the expiry period.

8 What is financial planning? Give the essential characters/ principles of financial planning. (S. 04)

☞ **Financial Planning**

"Financial planning is a process of deciding the financial activity required for an organisation to achieve predefined target and goals."

Features/Characteristics or Essentials of Financial Planning

1. It should be simple.
2. It should be changeable as per the needs.
3. It should give maximum returns to money.
4. It should prevent the unwanted expenditure.
5. It should have long foresight.
6. It should have the provisions of emerging funds.
7. It should be such that borrowing should be at minimum rate of interest.
8. It should have proper inventory for raw materials and official requirements.
9. It should have arrangement of sufficient funds for the sales department.
10. It should maintain proper stock of raw materials and finished products.
11. There should be proper control over activities of business as per financial planning.

12. It should be able to face or overcome the uncertain conditions like fire, flood, penalties, etc.

9 What is the importance or objectives of financial planning? (W. 05)

☞ **Objectives of Financial Planning**

1. To provide adequate funds to the business.
2. To create confidence amongest the investors.
3. To ensure fair return on investment.
4. To have a proper inventory of raw materials and finished product.
5. To decide the policy for best utilization of funds.
6. To develop and maintain proper relations with bank, financial institutes, workers and members of organisation.

10 Define share. Explain different types or kinds of shares.

☞ **Share**

When the capital is divided into smaller units then each unit is described as share.

Types of Share

a. Preference Share

• These shares carry preference regarding both dividend and the return of the capital.
• These shares are preferred by those people who do not like to risk their capital completely and want higher income than invested in other schemes.
• The preference shareholders gets a fixed dividend from the profits and the remaining profit is divided among the ordinary shareholders.
• The preference shareholders get a fixed dividend in case of winding up of the organisation.

b. Ordinary Shares (Equity Shares)

• The ordinary shareholders are the real owners of the organisation because the company is controlled by them.

- These shareholders have voting rights to elect the directors of the company.
- The dividend on these shares is paid after the dividend on the preference share has been paid.
- These shareholders have a risk because they get their claim only after the clearance of other claims.
- These shareholders are generally paid a higher rate of dividend.
- The rate of dividend on such shares depends upon the amount of profits available and the policy of the directors of the company in this regard.

Introduction to Accountancy

1 Define the terms. (S. 98, 00, 04, 05; W. 99, 05)

☞(a) **Account:** It is a systematically summarised record of all daily financial transactions.

(b) **Accountancy/accounting:** It is an art of recording, classifying, summarising the business transactions which helps in summarising records and finding out profits and losses.

(c) **Transaction:** Transaction is an event in which there is exchange of goods or services, in cash or on credit.

(d) **Capital:** It is the amount contributed by proprietor or partner in the business.

(e) **Asset:** Assets means cash and fixed properties of the business.

(f) **Liability:** It is the total amount or responsibilities payable by the business.

(g) **Creditor:** A person who gives something in cash or kind to another person is a creditor.

(h) **Debtor:** A person who receives something in cash or kind becomes debtor.

(i) **Solvency:** When total assets or business are more than or equal to liabilities, the condition is known as solvency.

(j) **Insolvency:** It is the condition in which liabilities are more than assets.

(k) **Drawings:** It is the amount of money withdrawn by owner from business to meet personal expenses.

(l) **Expenses:** Expenses are the efforts made by business to obtain revenues.

(m) **Revenue:** It represents accomplishment of the business.

(n) **Profit:** Profit is the excess of revenues over expenses in particular period.

(o) **Loss:** It is the excess expenses over income.

2 Give the objectives of accountancy.

☞ (i) It provides knowledge of all financial transactions.

(ii) It provides balances of creditors, debtors and expenses in different heads.

(iii) It provides information regarding total purchases, total sales, and closing stock.

(iv) It provides information to prepare profit and loss account and balance sheet.

(v) It provides total assets and liabilities of a concern.

3 What are the concepts of accountancy? (S. 08, 09; W. 04, 06)

☞(a) **Money measurement concept:** All the transactions in the books are recorded in terms of money. Nonfinancial events are not recorded.

(b) **Separate entity concept:** Business and businessman are two different entities. Recording of business transaction is done and not that of businessman.

(c) **Dual aspect concept:** Every transaction has got two entries. One is that of debit and other is credit. Both are equal in amount.

(d) **Going concern concept:** As per the concept, the life of business is infinite.

(e) **Accounting period concept:** Accounts are maintained for 12 months and preserved for future.

(f) **Cost concept:** The value of closing stock is always determined at cost price.

(g) **Actual event concept:** An entry is to be recorded in books only when an event takes place.

(h) **Matching concept:** It states that expenses in an accounting period should match with revenues in the period.

4 **Define bookkeeping. Give objectives and importance of bookkeeping. (S. 96, 98, 01, 08, 09; W. 99, 00)**

☞ **Bookkeeping**

"Bookkeeping is an art of recording business transactions in a regular and systematic manner."

Objectives of Bookkeeping

(a) **Primary objectives:**
    (i) To have a systematic record.
    (ii) To know profits or losses.
    (iii) To know financial position of business.

(b) **Secondary objectives:**
    (i) To know capital invested.
    (ii) To understand cash and stock at hand.
    (iii) To know creditors.
    (iv) To know debtors from whom bills are receivable.

(c) **Other objectives:**
    (i) To prevent mistakes, errors and frauds.
    (ii) To review progress of business.
    (iii) To provide information from time to time for decision making.

Importance of Bookkeeping

1. Bookkeeping is an art of recording, classifying and summarising business transactions, which provides correct information to businessman.
2. Bookkeeping and accountancy is important aspect of modern business for making policies and future plans.
3. Bookkeeping plays an important role in preparation of balance sheet.
4. Bookkeeping plays an important role in understanding the progress of a firm.
5. Bookkeeping is useful to know profits and losses of business.

5 **What do you mean by "double entry bookkeeping"? Give its advantages and disadvantages. (S. 96, 04, 07, 09; W. 96, 97, 00, 01)**

☞ **Double Entry Bookkeeping**

It is a method of bookkeeping based on a typical principle in which every transaction has two entries, i.e. creditor and debtor.

Advantages

1. The method is most reliable as it is based on some principle.
2. It is universally accepted method.
3. It provides arithmetic accuracy.
4. Information regarding any transaction can be obtained at any time.
5. This method records all possible effects of a business transaction.
6. Due to double entry, chances of frauds are minimum.
7. It helps in calculating profit/loss in any period.
8. The progress of business can be observed by making comparison of previous years.

Disadvantages

1. Detection of errors in original records becomes difficult.
2. Posting under wrong account head but on the right may remain undetected.
3. Omission of a transaction from recording cannot be found out easily.

6 **Differentiate between double entry system and single entry system.**

☞

Double entry system	Single entry system
1. It records each and every transaction of business.	1. It does not record all transactions.
2. Profit and loss can be calculated easily.	2. Profit and loss cannot be calculated in this method.
3. Balance sheet gives correct financial position.	3. Balance sheet cannot be prepared and thus financial position is not known.

Contd.

Double entry system	Single entry system
4. Personal, real and nominal accounts are maintained.	4. Only personal accounts are maintained.
5. Double entry gives accuracy.	5. It is not possible.
6. Comparisons are possible with previous periods.	6. Comparisons are not possible with previous periods.
7. Errors and frauds can be detected.	7. It is not easy to detect errors and frauds.

7 Mention the advantages of accountancy/accounting.

☞ *a. Advantages for Traders*

1. It removes limitations of human memory.
2. It gives a clear picture with reasons and proofs about the profits and losses.
3. It helps in knowing present market value of business.
4. It helps in calculating amount receivable and amounts payable.
5. It helps in comparing financial results over several years.
6. It helps in tax calculation.
7. The books can be provided as a proof in the court of law.

b. Advantages for Government

1. For tax calculation.
2. As a source of information about employment in country.

c. Advantages for Suppliers, Creditors and Shareholders

They can modify the decision by knowing business position.

8 Define account. Give types/classification of accounts. (S. 05, 08, 09; W. 02)

☞ **Account**

It is a systematically summarised record of all daily financial transactions.

Types/Classification

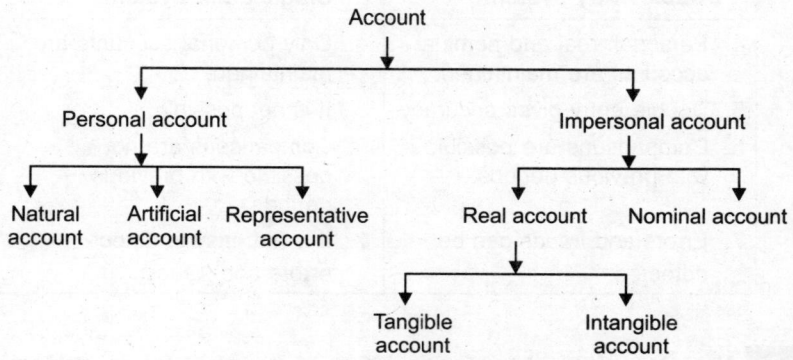

A. Personal Account

It is the account of individual firms, local authorities, associations as well as creditors or debtors.

(a) **Natural account:** Name of the person is recorded.

(b) **Artificial account:** Firms, associations, local authorities which exist legally.

(c) **Representative account:** Debtors, creditors A/c.

B. Impersonal Account

It is not related to particular person or names.

(a) **Real account:** It is related to assets or properties of the business.

(i) *Tangible account:* It is the account related to assets or properties which can be seen or touched or measured, e.g. land, building, cash, etc.

(ii) *Intangible account:* It is related to the assets which cannot be seen, touched and measured, e.g. goodwill, patent rights, copyrights, advertisements.

(b) **Nominal account:** Nominal account is item of expenses, incomes and gains, discounts and salary.

9 Define 'accounting conventions'. Explain various conventions commonly used in preparation of accounting statements.

☞ The customs which must be followed in accountancy while preparing the accounting statements are termed as accounting conventions.

Various Conventions

(a) **Convention of full disclosure:** The financial statement should disclose the information 'fully and fairly'. As per Indian Companies Act, the final account of company must give a true and fair picture of affairs of company.

(b) **Convention of consistancy:** It states that accounting practices should remain unchanged from one period to another period.

(c) **Convention of conservation:** It states that 'anticipate, 'no profit' and provide for all possible losses. As per this convention, liabilities are recorded first and revenues are recognised later.

(d) **Convention of materiality:** Only those transactions are recorded which influence significantly.

(e) **Convention of objectivity:** The records should be free from personal feelings and judgements.

Cash Book

1 **Define cash book. Give objectives and types of cash book. (S. 96, 97, 99, 01, 02, 03, 08; W. 96, 97, 01, 04)**

☞ **Cash Book**

Cash book is the book of accounts in which all the cash transactions are recorded and maintained.

Objectives of Cash Book

1. To save the time in preparing journal and ledger.
2. To collect and record all the cash transactions.
3. To calculate cash at hand.
4. To save the workers engenged in maintaining records.

Types of Cash Book

1. Single column cash book.
2. Double column cash book.
3. Triple column cash book.
4. Petty cash book: It is of two types:
    (i) Simple petty cash book.
    (ii) Analytical petty cash book.

2 **Define the terms. (S. 02)**

☞ **Contra entry**

Contra entry are those which do not require their posting into ledger. The 'C' is marked after the entry to avoid any mistake during ledgering.

Imprest System

It is the system followed in petty cash book. In this system, the cashier hands over a fixed amount to the petty cashier at the beginning of a week or month. This amount is called imprest amount. The petty cashier submits the accounts of petty cash to the cashier at the end of week or month. The cashier recovers the expenses made by the petty cashier.

3 **Write a note on petty cash book. (S. 98, 99, 01, 02, 08, 09; W. 96, 97, 98, 99, 03, 04)**

☞ **Petty Cash Book**

It is the book of account which records the transactions of minor amounts (petty) and those transactions which are essentially take place on cash basis.

Examples

Stationary, cooliage, telephone, travelling, etc. In large organisations a person is appointed to make minor cash payments. He is known as petty cashier. The petty cashier receives a definite amount from cashier and he uses the same in a definite period (7 days, 15 days, 30 days, etc. At the end of the period, petty cashier submits the records and the cash balance to the cashier. The cashier recovers the expenses made to the petty cashier. This is known as "imprest system".

1. **Simple petty cash book:** It is similar to general cash book having two sides receipts and payments.

Simple Petty Cash Book

Receipts Rs	CBF	Date	Particulars	V No.	Payments Rs

2. **Analytical petty cash book (columnar petty cash book):** In this type, receipts are recorded on right side. The left side has two columns for the amount received and the cash book folio (CBF) number, with date and particulars. Payment side is suitably analysed into columns for entering in various types of expenses.

Analytical Petty Cash Book

Receipts Rs	CBF	Date	Particulars	V No.	Payments Rs	Post and Telephone	Coolie	Travelling

Journal, Ledger and Trial Balance

1 **Define journal. Give importance/utility of journal. Give format of journal. (S. 96, 02, 03, 06, 08; W. 98, 01, 02)**

☞ **Journal**

" A journal is a book of original entries in which all the transactions are recorded in chronological order."

Utility/Importance

1. It contains record of all transactions.
2. As it is the first book, it provides all information about every transaction.
3. It helps in locating errors.
4. It saves time in preparation of other records.
5. It has legal standing.

Format of Journal

Date	Particulars	Bill No.	LF No.	Amount			
				Debit		Credit	
				Rs	Ps	Rs	Ps
Year/	....A/c...Dr			xxx	xx		
Day/	To....A/c...Cr					xx	xxx
Month	(Being...)						
				Total		Total	

Explanation

(a) **Date column:** In the date column, the year is written at the top and for every transaction the month and day are entered.

(b) **Particulars:** Name of the account to be debited is written. 'Dr.' is written after it. On the next line name of the amount to be credited is written. The prefix used is 'To'. The narration is written in bracket. The prefix is "Being" A closing line is drawn in the column after every transaction.

(c) **Bill number:** The number on the bill is entered, it facilitates the cross check.

(d) **LF number:** It is the ledger folio number. The page number on which the account is separated in a ledger is written.

(e) **Amount:** Amount column is divided into debit and credit amount. Both should be written on the same line. At the end of the page and after entering all the transactions the total of debit and credit amounts are calculated.

2 **Define ledger. Give its importance. Give format of ledger. (S. 96, 97, 98, 99, 02, 04; W. 98, 99, 01)**

☞ **Ledger**

"Ledger is the book of original entries prepared from journal, in which one page or more pages are devoted to a particular account and contains records of all personal, real and nominal accounts."

The ledger can be maintained in a bound register or loose leaflets.

Objectives

(i) To have summary of journal.

(ii) To find out final position of any account.

(iii) To calculate total amount payable.

(iv) To calculate total amount receivable.

Importance of Ledger in Double Entry Bookkeeping

(i) It provides the information under different heads like assets, liabilities, income, expenses and losses.

(ii) Profit and loss A/c can easily be prepared with the help of ledger account.

(iii) Balance sheet is also prepared with the help of ledger A/cs.

Format of Ledger

Dr.   **Name of A/c.......**   Cr.

Date	Parti-culars	JF No.	Amount	Date	Parti-cular	JF No.	Amount
Year Month Day	To Goods A/c			Y/M/D	By.... A/c		
			Total				Total

Explanation

There are two halves namely 'Debit' and 'Credit' sides.

(i) The name of A/c is written at the top in block letters.

(ii) **Date:** The date should be written in a sequence like year, month and day.

(iii) **Particulars:** In this column, the name of account affected is written and prefix 'To' is used on debit side and 'By' on credit side.

(iv) **JF number:** It is the page number in journal from which the ledger is prepared.

(v) **Amount:** The entries are made accordingly.

3 "Ledger is the principal book of accounts in business". Explain. (S. 99, 08)

☞ Because:

(i) Every entry made in journal must be posted into the ledger.

(ii) Every entry should be posted in debit as well as credit A/c.

(iii) Ledger gives the information related to the particular person or head.

(iv) The ledger has an account for every person, thing or item of profit and loss, income, etc.

(v) Profit and loss A/c can be prepared by ledger.

(vi) Balance sheet can be prepared by ledger.

Thus, it shows that "ledger is the principal book of accounts in business".

4 Differentiate between journal and ledger. (S. 99, 05, 06)

☞

Journal	Ledger
1. It is a book of original entry.	1. It is a book of secondary entry.
2. It is a book for chronological record, i.e. the transactions are recorded as and when they take place.	2. It is the book for analytical record, i.e. all the transactions relating to particular account are recorded in order of their occurrence.
3. Balancing is not done.	3. All the accounts are balanced.
4. From the journal, entries are transferred to ledger.	4. From the ledger, the trial balance is drawn and then financial statements are prepared from it.
5. The unit of classification of data within the journal is transaction.	5. The unit of classification of data within the ledger is account.
6. The process of recording entries in the journal is called "journalising".	6. The process of recording entries in the ledger is called "posting".

5 What is trial balance? Give its objectives/importance. (S. 96, 97, 98, 02, 03, 06, 08; W. 98, 99, 00, 01, 02, 03, 04)

☞ **Trial Balance**

"The trial balance is the statement of debit and credit balances extracted from ledger, with a view to test arithmetical accuracy of the books."

Objectives

1. To check principles of double entry bookkeeping.
2. To check arithmetical accuracy of journal and ledger.
3. To provide information from time to time to the management.
4. To help in preparation of final account.
5. To check the entries of transactions in the books.

6 **What are different methods of preparation of trial balance? (S. 97, 02, 09; W. 00, 01, 03, 04, 06)**

☞ **Methods of Trial Balance**

1. **Total method:** In this method, all names of ledger A/c are written. The total of the A/c (debit and credit total) before balancing the ledger are entered.

Name of A/c	LF No.	Debit total amount	Credit total amount
		Total	Total

2. **Balance method:** In this method, balance is brought down on the opposite sides of the accounts. "To balance c/d" is written on the debit side and "By balance b/d" is written on credit side.

Name of A/c	LF No.	Debit balance amount	Credit balance amount
		Total	Total

3. **Total and balance method:**

Name of A/c	LF No.	Debit total amount	Credit total amount	Debit amount balance	Credit balance amount
		1	2	3	4

Total of 1 = Total of 2,   Total of 3 = Total of 4

7 **What are the errors observed in trial balance? OR Explain disclosed errors (affected) and undisclosed errors (not affected/not reflected) in trial balance statement. (S. 96; W. 02, 03)**

☞ **a. Disclosed Errors**

Definition: "The errors which affect or reflect the trial balance are called disclosed errors."

Examples/Reasons for Disclosed Errors

1. Posting of wrong amount in the ledger from the journal, the trial balance will not agree.
2. Wrong totaling of ledger books would affect the trial balance.
3. Omission of a ledger account in a trial balance.
4. Duplication of entry.
5. Posting of entry on the wrong side will affect the trial balance.
6. Wrong balancing of ledger accounts.

b. Undisclosed Errors

Definition: "The errors which do not affect or not reflect the trial balance are called undisclosed errors."

Examples

1. Omission of an entry in the books of original entry will not affect trial balance.
2. Recording wrong amount in the books of original entry.
3. Considering wrong amount of a transaction in journal will affect the journal.
4. **Compensating errors:** These are the errors which are neutralised by making entry of same amount on credit side and debit side but in different heads.

Final Accounts

1 **Define final accounts. Give its types. (W. 96, 98)**

☞ **Final Account/Statement**

" Final accounts are financial statements which give complete picture of business at the end of accounting period."

Types of Final Accounts

1. Income statement:
    (i) Trading account
    (ii) Profit and loss account
2. Balance sheet.

2 **Define trading account. Give its format.**

☞ **Trading Account**

"It is the part of income statement prepared to know amounts of "gross profit" or "gross loss" during a particular time period".

Format of Trading Account

Trading A/c of _____
For the period ending on _____
                    Dr.   Cr.

Particulars	Amount	Particulars	Amount
To opening stock A/c	xxx	By sales A/c	
To purchase A/c....		Cash sales	xxx

Contd.

Particulars	Amount	Particulars	Amount
Cash purchase	xxx	Credit sales	xxx
Credit purchase	xxx	Sales return	xxx
Purchase return	xxx	By closing stock	xxx
To direct expenses			
To carriage A/c	xxx		
To coolie charges	xxx		
To octroi	xxx		
To wages	xxx		
To gross profit c/d	xxx	By gross loss c/d	xxx
To gross loss b/d	xxx	By gross profit b/d	xxx

3 Define "profit and loss account". Give specimen format. (S. 98, 99, 01, 03; W. 97, 98, 99, 00, 01, 03, 04)

☞ **Profit and Loss Account**

"It is the part of income statement prepared to know " net profit" and "net loss" during particular period of time."

Format of Profit and Loss Account

Profit and loss A/c of _____

For the period ending on _____

Dr.   Cr.

Particulars	Amount	Particulars	Amount
To gross loss b/d	xxx	By gross profit b/d	xxx
To office expenses	xxx		
To salary	xxx	By commission received	xxx
To salaries and wages	xxx	By rent received	xxx
To rent and taxes	xxx	By interest as investment	xxx
To postage and telephone	xxx	By discount received	xxx

Contd.

Particulars	Amount	Particulars	Amount
To printing and stationary	xxx	By interest on drawings	xxx
To selling expenses	xxx		
To advertisement	xxx		
To commission to salesman	xxx		
To finantial expenses	xxx		
To repair and maintenance	xxx		
To legal charges	xxx		
To accounting fees	xxx		
To finance expenses	xxx		
To expenses to loss of goods and fire	xxx		
To net profit c/d		**By net loss c/d**	

Importance of Profit and Loss Account

1. It is prepared to find out amount of net profit earned in the year.
2. Profit and loss account is a summary of all indirect expenses related to office administration, selling and distribution and financing the business.

4 Define balance sheet. Give format of balance sheet. (S. 96, 98, 99, 01, 02, 03, 04, 07, 09; W. 96, 97, 99, 00, 01, 04)

☞ Balance Sheet

"A balance sheet is a statement of the financial position of a business on a given date."Or
"A balance sheet is a statement of assets and liabilities of a business on a particular date."

Format of Balance Sheet

Balance sheet of _____
For the period ending on _____

Liabilities	Amount	Assets	Amount
Fixed liabilities		Fixed assets	
Long-term loans	xxx	Land	xxx
+ Interest on capital	xxx	Building	xxx
+ Net profit	xxx	Machinery	xxx
– Net loss	xxx	Furniture	xxx
– Drawing	xxx	Tools	xxx
Current liabilities	xxx	Vehicles	xxx
Bank over drafts	xxx	Bank deposits	xxx
Sundry creditors	xxx	Cash at bank	xxx
Bills payable	xxx	Temporary investment	xxx
Outstanding expenses	xxx	Sundry debtors	xxx
Income received in		Advertisement	xxx
advance	xxx	Copyright, patents	xxx
		Finished goods	xxx
		Raw materials	xxx
		Semifinished goods	xxx
	Total		**Total**

5 Define assets and give classification of assets. (W. 96, 98, 01)

☞ **Assets**

"Assets are the properties of every description owned by the business."

1. **Fixed assets:** They are permanent assets. They are the long-term assets of the business, e.g. land, building, plant, machinery, furniture, equipment.
2. **Current assets (floating assets):** They are the assets which are having a definite life (1 to 3 years). Current assets include cash and any other assets that are easily converted into cash within a short period of time usually a year, e.g. bank deposits, investment.
3. **Liquid assets:** They are the properties which are consumed at any time, e.g. cash at hand, cash at bank, temporary investment, sundry debtor.

4. **Fictitious assets (intangible assets):** Their role can be measured directly. They can neither be touched nor seen hence called intangible assets, e.g. advertisement, copyright, patents, goodwill.

5. **Tangible assets:** The assets which can be touched and seen are called tangible assets, e.g. land, building, machinery, furniture.

6 Define liabilities. Give the classification of liabilities. (W. 96, 98)

☞ **Liabilities**

Liabilities are the debts of the business.

Classification

1. **Fixed liabilities:** Those which should be paid over a long period, e.g. long-term loans, capital.

2. **Current liabilities:** These are payable in a period less than one year, e.g. short-term loans, over drafts, bills payable, sundry creditors.

3. **Contingent liabilities:** These are not the liabilities at present but can occur in future, e.g. contingencies like legal penalties, worker compensation, etc.

7 Differentiate between the following: (S. 05, 08)

☞	Profit and loss account	Balance sheet
	1. In profit and loss account the nominal accounts are shown.	1. In balance sheet personal account and real accounts are shown.
	2. The aim of profit and loss account is to provide information regarding "net profit" and "net loss".	2. The aim of balance sheet is to know the financial position of the business.
	3. It is a ledger account giving information about debit and credits.	3. It is only statement of asset and liabilities.
	4. It is an account, so the words 'To' and 'By' are used.	4. It is a statement and the words 'To' and 'By' are not used.

Contd.

Profit and loss account	Balance sheet
5. The balance of the profit and loss accounts indicates profit or loss.	5. The total of both sides of a balance sheet is always the same.
6. The accounts show a profit or loss made by business as on a fixed date.	6. It shows the financial position of the business enterprises on a fixed date.

Trial balance	Balance sheet
1. Trial balance is a statement of debit or credit balances extracted from ledger with a view to test arithmetical accuracy of books.	1. Balance sheet is a statement of accounts prepared for the purpose of measuring the exact financial position of business on the last date of financial year.
2. The aim of trial balance is to provide information regarding accuracy of books.	2. The aim of balance sheet is to know financial position of business.
3. It is the ledger account giving information about debits and credits.	3. It is only statement of assets and liabilities.
4. It is an account so the words 'To' and 'By' are used.	4. It is a statement and words 'To' and 'By' are not used.
5. The balance of profit and loss account indicates profit and loss.	5. The total on both sides of balance sheet is always the same.
6. The account shows profit or loss made by the business as on a fixed date.	6. It shows the financial position of the business on a fixed date.

Analysis of Financial Statements

1 **Define financial analysis. What are different methods used for financial analysis? How is financial analysis carried out? (S. 97, 98, 05, 07, 08, 09; W. 97, 98, 00, 02, 04)**

☞ **Financial Analysis**

"It means the systematic classification, comparison and examination of the facts and figures as disclosed in the statement to have full knowledge regarding the profitability and financial position of the company."

Methods of Financial Analysis

a. Comparative Financial Statement

In this method, the data over at least 2 accounting periods is placed side by side and comparison of performance of business over the year is done. It helps in judging future course of activities. Comparative income statements and comparative balance sheets are published by large organisations for the interest of outsiders.

b. Common Size Financial Statement

These are the statements in which given figures are converted into % figures on some basis, e.g.

  1. Figures in sales in trading A/c are taken as 100%.
  2. In balance sheet either total assets or total liabilities are taken as 100% and remaining figures are calculated.

c. Trend Analysis

The method is combination of comparative and common size statement.

In this method, figures in final statement of one of the past years (base year) are taken as 100. All the remaining figures in that year and next years are converted accordingly and published.

d. Ratio Analysis

A ratio expresses the relationship between 2 items of financial statement. It may be defined as relation between two accounting figures expressed in mathematical terms.

Advantages of Ratio Analysis

1. Easy to calculate and understand.
2. Easy to compare.
3. Easy to interpret.
4. Indicates trends and efficiency of organisation.
5. Helps in future planning.

Disadvantages (Limitations) of Ratio Analysis

1. Ratio will be misleading if information in final account is misleading, improper or falsified.
2. The ratio analysis explains the past and not the future.
3. Interpretation is difficult.
4. Inter-firm comparison is possible only if both firms are adopting same procedure.
5. Implementation of accounting method must be uniform in the life of business.

2 Define the term 'ratio'. Give the classification of ratios.

☞ Ratio

A ratio is the relationship between two accounting figures expressed in mathematical terms.

Classification of Ratios

(a) Liquidity ratios
(b) Activity ratios
(c) Solvency or leverage ratios
(d) Profitability ratios

(a) Liquidity ratios

They indicate the capacity of business to pay off its liabilities in time. They are calculated by

(a) Current ratios $= \dfrac{\text{Current assets}}{\text{Current liabilities}}$

Standard 2:1 or more is expected.

(b) Quick ratio $= \dfrac{\text{Quick asset}}{\text{Current liabilities}}$

(c) Liquid ratio $= \dfrac{\text{Liquid asset}}{\text{Current liabilities}}$

Standard 1:1 or more is expected.

(d) Absolute liquid ratio $= \dfrac{\text{Absolute liquid asset}}{\text{Current liabilities}}$

Standard 0.5:1 or more is expected.

(b) Activity ratios

Turnover ratios/efficiency ratios

It measures efficiency of business with which it uses its resources or assets.

(a) Inventory turnover ratio: It is also known as stock turnover ratio.

It gives the firm inventory management.

Inventory turnover ratio $= \dfrac{\text{Cost of goods sold}}{\text{Average inventory}}$

   (i) A higher inventory turnover ratio indicates under investment in inventory. It creates risk of "out of stock".

  (ii) A low inventory turnover ratio indicates over investment in inventory which results in high costs.

(b) Capital turnover ratio: This ratio indicates relationship between sales and the capital employed in business.

(c) Inventory conversion period: It measures the ability of business to convert invertory into finished goods.

$$\text{ICP} = \dfrac{\text{Average stock}}{\text{Cost of goods sold}} \times \text{Number of working days}$$

(c) Solvency ratios (S. 02)
They indicate ability of business to meet long-term requirement.

(a) Debit equity ratio = $\dfrac{\text{Total debt}}{\text{Total equity}}$

(b) Long-term equity ratio = $\dfrac{\text{Long-term debts}}{\text{Total equity}}$

(d) Profitability ratios
They measure profitability.

(a) Gross profitability ratio: It establishes relationship of gross profit with net sales.

Gross profit ratio = $\dfrac{\text{Gross profit}}{\text{Net sales}} \times 100$

(b) Overall profitability ratio:

Return on assets = $\dfrac{\text{Net profit after taxes}}{\text{Total asset}} \times 100$

(c) Net profit ratio: This ratio is also known as net profit margin. It gives the relationship between net profit and net sales.

Net profit ratio = $\dfrac{\text{Net profit}}{\text{Total sales}} \times 100$

3 Give the importance/objectives of financial analysis/ analysis of financial statements. (S. 03)

☞ 1. To know nature and extent of assest and liabilities
2. To find out the profit
3. To find out the liquidity
4. To find out whether the firm is doing well
5. To find out solvency
6. To find out the financial and credit position
7. To calculate various ratios
8. To calculate the taxes to be paid
9. To have plan for future
10. To make comparison with past
11. To provide efficient operation.

Budget and Budgeting

1 Define the terms. (S. 96, 97, 01, 02, 04, 07; W. 97, 98, 99, 01, 02, 04)

☞ **Budget:** "A budget is a written statement of planned activities of a firm for a definite period of time."

Budgetary period: "The period for which the plan of budget is prepared is termed as budget period."

Budgetary control: "It means the process of constant checking and evolution of actual result achieved as compared with budget goals."

2 What are the main objectives of budgetary control? (S. 96, 97, 01, 04; W. 97, 98, 99, 02, 05)

☞ The main objectives of budgetary control are:

a. Planning

- A budget is a plan of action.
- It involves plans for production, sale target, etc.
- The proper planning of budget will give progress of the firm.

b. Coordination

Coordination is the process of cooperation between divisions of a concern work.

- An effective coordination requires proper communication of objectives and instructions.

- For better coordination, the copies of budget plan should be given to all management personnels.

c. **Control**

- Control is the action necessary for implementation of plan and to achieve the goal.
- Proper reporting of any sort of changes in the budget plan should be informed to management for its corrective action.

3 Give advantages and disadvantages of budgetary control. (S. 99, 02, 07, 08; W. 96, 99)

☞ **Budgetary Control**

Advantages

1. It brings efficiency in working of business.
2. It coordinates activities in all departments.
3. It offers centralised control by decentralizing responsibilities.
4. It minimizes wastages and losses.
5. It facilitates comparison of actual work with past.
6. It facilitates appropriate financing.
7. It assures safety to management and creditor.
8. It utilises the full plant capacities and manpower.

Disadvantages

1. A resistance may be observed from workers.
2. Uncertain market conditions may prove the budgetary control meaningless.
3. If excess time is spent in budget preparation, it becomes less important.
4. It requires continuous supervision.
5. As it is a teamwork, coordination has greatest importance. Any miscoordination is not tolerated.

4 Give the limitations of budgetary control. (S. 97, 08; W. 03, 04)

☞1. Budget control does not replace the management but infact it is a tool of management.
2. The strength and weakness of budget depend on the efficient working or implementation of plan.

3. The budget preparation requires a long experience for correct realisation of budgetary goals.

4. Budgetary operations become very costly and thus co-relations between the cost and budgetary operations should be considered.

5 Mention the fuctions of budget committee. (S. 03)

☞ 1. To provide past data for deciding future plans.
2. To issue instructions for budget requirements.
3. To give general policies of the budget.
4. To advise regarding preparation of budget.
5. To take approval from the different departments.
6. To suggest revisions and amendments to budgets.
7. To approve budgets.
8. To prepare budget summaries, if required.
9. To prepare the master budget.
10. To receive study and analyse periodical reports.
11. To consider recommendations from different departments.

6 What are requirements of effective budgeting/budgetary control? (W. 05)

☞ A successful budgeting programme can be carried out only with following coordinations:

1. Budgeting must have the complete cooperation of top management.
2. There should be an accurate accounting system.
3. Budget should be prepared with the knowledge of the business policy to be adopted during the period.
4. An effective system of budgetary control requires vigilance at all levels.
5. Budget committee must include officers from all the departments of the organisation for proper and successful implementation of the budget.
6. The budget system should not cost more to operate than it is worth.
7. Budget should be practically possible to gain maximum profit.

7 Give the classification of budget. (S. 08; W. 04)

☞

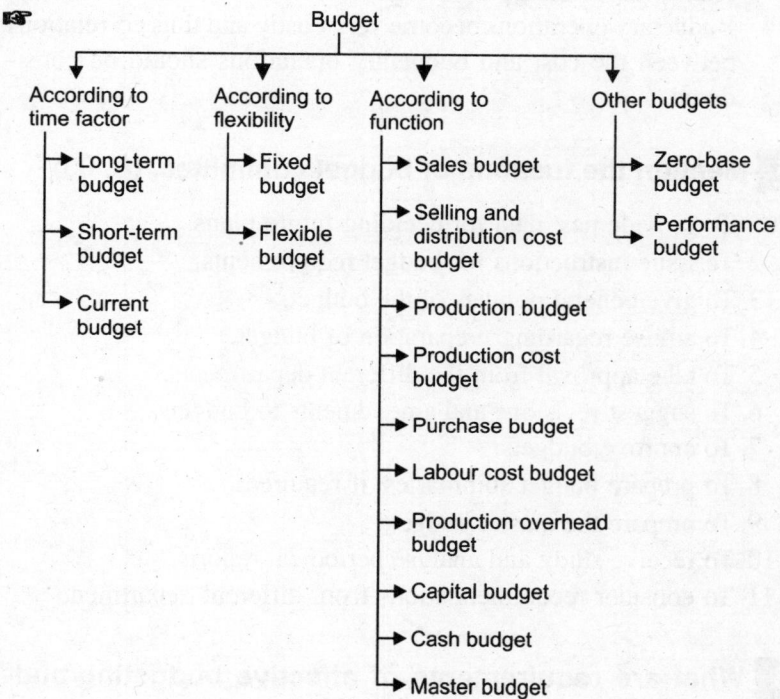

(a) According to Time Factor

(a) Long-term budget: Budget is prepared for a period of 5 to 10 years.
(b) Short-term budget: Budget is prepared for a period 1 to 2 years.
(c) Current budget: Budget is prepared for period of 1 month.

(b) According to Flexibility

(a) Fixed budget: In this type, once the budget is fixed there is no any change.
(b) Flexible budget: It is designed to change accordingly to actually required. It is more elastic, useful and practical. As per the need, budget can be increased.

(c) According to Function

A functional budget is one which relates to any of the functions of organisation.

(i) Sales budget

(ii) Purchase budget

(iii) Production budget

(iv) Capital budget

(v) Production cost budget

(vi) Cash budget.

(d) Other Budgets

(i) *Zero-Base Budget*

- It does not mean that there should not be any increase or decrease in activities over past years.
- In zero-base budget, zero is taken as a starting point (base) and budget is developed on the basis of likely activities for future period.
- The concept originated in USA in 1970.
- It requires closer participation of all managers and removal of communication gap to reduce cost along with revenue generation.

(ii) *Performance Budget*

- This type originated in USA in 1947 to prove accounting in USA.
- In performance budget, "purpose of objectives for which funds are required is presented".
- It also includes costs of programmes proposed and quantitative data measuring fulfilment of work; so, in other words, the more importance is given to output than to input.
- For better implementation, it requires segmentation of organisation, understanding roles by every segment and planned execution of work.

Board Question Papers

(From Summer 1996 to Summer 2017)

Summer Examination 1996
D Pharm Second Year
Drug Store and Business Management

Q 1. Solve any *five* of the following:

a. Define the term business.

b. Define the term partnership. List out merits and demerits of partnership.

c. Define the terms:

    i. Trial balance   ii. Balance sheet

d. Give the main objectives of cash book.

e. Define the term budget and why budgetary control is necessary.

f. What is safety stock and inventory carrying cost?

Q 2. Solve any *four* of the following:

a. Define the term aids to trade. Discuss important aids to trade.

b. Write short note on elements of economics.

c. Match the following:

    i. Business means:
- Trade and commerce
- Buying and selling goods
- Commerce
- Industry and commerce

    ii. "The buying and selling of goods in order to make profit is called:"
- Trade
- Direct services
- Indirect services
- Commerce

d. Define cooperative organization. Give its advantages and disadvantages.

e. i. A wholesaler acts as a link between manufacturer and:
   - Retailer
   - Consumers
   - Both (1) and (2)
   - Neither (1) nor (2)

   ii. Wholesalers should be removed from the chain of distribution because they:
   - Provide services to producers
   - Help in increasing the product
   - Provide services to retailer
   - Increase the price of the goods

Q 3. Solve any *four* of the following:

a. What do you mean by purchasing? What are its essentials?

b. Explain in brief what do you mean by:
   i. Tender   ii. Contract

c. What are the factors to be taken into consideration for the selection of suppliers?

d. Name various forms of business organization. Write a note on any one of them with its advantages.

e. Write short note on 'codification of drugs'.

Q 4. Solve any *four* of the following:

a. Discuss the objectives and importance of inventory control.

b. What do you mean by Economic Order Quantity (EOQ)?

c. Explain importance of VED analysis.

d. Explain what do you mean by maximum and minimum stock level.

e. Explain the procedure to be followed for the disposal of surplus stock.

Q 5. Solve any *four* of the following:

a. What do you understand by market research? Explain its objectives.

b. How is salesmanship important for business?

c. Window display is one of the forms of advertisement. Explain.

d. What is general ledger, how is it maintained?

e. Explain the terms profit and loss account and balance sheet.

Q 6. Solve any *four* of the following:

a. Discuss in short importance of different kinds of accounts.

b. Define bookkeeping. What are various advantages of bookkeeping.

c. What are the various advantages of double entry bookkeeping.

d. Explain the term general ledger. Distinguish between journal and ledger.

e. Discuss the different methods of preparation of 'trial balance'. State various errors which are not disclosed by trial balance.

Winter Examination 1996
D Pharm Second Year
Drug Store and Business Management

Q 1. Solve any *five* of the following:

a. Define the term "cash book".

b. State importance of advertising.

c. State different types of bank accounts.

d. Define the terms:
    i. Asset   ii. Liabilities

e. What do you mean by "petty cash book"?

f. State what do you mean by final accounts.

Q 2. Solve any *four* of the following:

a. Give functions and subdivisions of commerce.

b. State element of 'economics and management'.

c. How will you select site of a drug store? What do you mean by layout of drug store?

d. What do you mean by purchasing? Give its importance. Give the objectives of purchasing.

e. What are various forms of business organization? Write a note on partnership.

Q 3. Solve any *four* of the following:

a. What do you mean by codification of drugs? What are its advantages?

b. What do you mean by tender? Explain various types of tenders.

c. Write short note on 'bank-credit facility'.

d. Discuss the importance and objectives of inventory control.

e. Define the following terms:
    i. Minimum stock level   iii. VED analysis
    ii. Maximum stock level   iv. Lead time

Q 4. Solve any *four* of the following:

a. What do you mean by EOQ (Economic Order Quantity). Give the importance in inventory control.

b. What are various channels of distribution of drugs?

c. Enlist the good qualities of a salesman.

d. Write a short note on "window-display".

e. What is market research? How does market research help for evaluation of sales promotion?

Q 5. Solve any *four* of the following:

a. Write in brief about recruitment and training of pharmacist.

b. Discuss in brief sources of finance.

c. List out kinds of bank accounts. What are the advantages of current account?

d. Give importance of finance in business.

e. What do you mean by bookkeeping? What are the objectives of bookkeeping.

Q 6. Solve any *four* of the following:

a. Define the terms:
   i. Account
   ii. Credit
   iii. Debit
   iv. Transaction
   v. Accounting

b. Discuss the main objectives of 'cash book'. State different types of cash book.

c. Write short note on bank reconciliation statement.

d. What is budgeting? State its importance.

e. Give an example of a typical profit and loss account and balance sheet of the business.

Summer Examination 1997
D Pharm Second Year
Drug Store and Business Management

Q 1. Solve any *five* of the following:

a. Define the terms:
   i. Industry
   ii. Commerce

b. What are the objectives of layout design of a drug store?

c. Define the term bank. List out the services offered by the bank.

d. Give objectives of inventory control.

e. What is market research? What are its objectives?

f. What is cash book?

g. State the importance of window display.

Q 2. Solve any *four* of the following:

a. Give the classification of various business activities.

b. Define the term trade. Give its classification.

c. Discuss various forms of business organization in short.

d. Discuss various kinds of partners in partnership form of business.

e. Elaborate the channels of distribution in pharmaceutical marketing.

Q 3. Solve any *four* of the following:

a. Define the following terms:

i. Lead time	iv. Maximum stock level
ii. Safety stock	v. Inventory carrying cost
iii. Minimum stock level	

b. How will you select site of a drug store? What do you mean by layout of drug store?

c. What do you mean by codification of drugs? What are its advantages? State various types of codification.

d. What is 'ABC' technique of inventory control?

e. What do you mean by tender? Explain various types of tender.

Q 4. Solve any *four* of the following:

a. Define the term budget. What do you mean by budgetary control?

b. Discuss various types of bank accounts. Give salient features of cheque.

c. Define the term finance. List out important sources of finance.

d. What is the principle of double entry book-keeping? Give its advantages.

e. Prepare a simple cash book from the following transactions and also prepare the necessary accounts in the ledger:

Year 1995	Particulars	Rs.
January 1	Cash in hand	10,000
January 2	Purchased machinery	4,000
January 3	Purchased furniture	1,000
January 6	Purchased building	4,000
January 7	Purchased goods for cash	1,000
January 15	Goods sold for cash	1,800
January 23	Paid salaries	300
January 27	Received from Akshay	1,000

Q 5. Solve any *four* of the following:
a. Explain the term ledger. Explain the different items in a specimen ledger.
b. Why is trial balance prepared? Discuss the different methods of preparations of trial balance.
c. Give an example of a typical profit and loss accout and balance sheet of the business.
d. What is VED analysis? State its importance.
e. What are commonly used means in analysing financial statements?

Q 6. Solve any *four* of the following:
a. Write short note on scrap and surplus disposal.
b. What do you mean by purchasing? Give its importance and objectives.
c. What is salesmanship? Enlist different qualities a salesman should possess.
d. What factors should be taken into consideration in evaluating the performance of a pharmacist?
e. Discuss various modes of training of a pharmacy personnel.
f. Write a note on "safety stock".

Summer Examination 1998
D Pharm Second Year
Drug Store and Business Management

Q 1. Solve any *five* of the following:
a. State different forms of business organizations.
b. Give elements of economics.
c. What is inventory control? Define the term lead time.
d. Define the following terms:
   i. Account   iii. Liabilities
   ii. Assets   iv. Capital
e. Enlist advantages and disadvantages of cooperative business organization.
f. What are the legal requirements and general conditions for opening a medical store?

Q 2. Solve any *four* of the following:
a. What is Joint Hindu Family business? Describe its main features.
b. Give short account on agreement of partnership deed.
c. Define the term trade. Enlist various aids to trade. Describe pharmaceutical advertisement.

    d. Define the terms commerce and management. What do you understand by pharmaceutical management?

    e. Mention advantages and disadvantages of channels of distribution. Mention the services of wholesalers.

Q 3. Solve any *four* of the following:

    a. Enlist methods of drugs codification. Give advantages of codification.

    b. How will you handle in general medical or drug store?

    c. What are the objectives of purchasing? Give the details of selection of supplier.

    d. Enlist the different documents required to open a new medical store.

    e. Give a typical layout of medical or drug store.

Q 4. Solve any *four* of the following:

    a. Mention different methods of inventory control. Give advantages of perpetual inventory control system.

    b. What do you understand by lead time and safety stock?

    c. Explain the minimum and maximum level of inventory. What is re-ordering level?

    d. Write short notes on:

        i. Economic order quantity   ii. VED analysis

    e. Give different methods of market research. What are advantages of market research?

Q 5. Solve any *two* of the following:

    a.   i. What do you mean by petty cash book? Illustrate it with suitable example.

       ii. What do you mean by:
- Cash-credit facility
- Object of crossing cheque
- Over-draft facility

    b.   i. Write a short account on financial management and financial planning.

       ii. What are different sources of finance available to business?

    c. Prepare a simple cash book from the following transactions and also prepare the necessary accounts in the ledger:

Year 1996	Particulars	Rs.
January 1	Cash in hand	10,000
January 2	Purchased machinery	4,000
January 3	Purchased furniture	1,000

Contd.

Year 1996	Particulars	Rs.
January 6	Purchased building	4,000
January 7	Purchased goods for cash	1,000
January 15	Goods sold for cash	1,800
January 23	Paid salaries	300
January 27	Received from Hemraj	1,000

Q 6. Solve any *two* of the following:

a.   i. Define the terms:
   - Journal
   - Trial balance
   - Ledger

    ii. Give the objectives of bookkeeping. What are the advantages of double entry bookkeeping?

b.   i. Define financial analysis. What are different methods used for financial analysis?

    ii. Mention object of preparing the trial balance. Mention the errors disclosed by trial balance.

c. Give the specimen format of profit and loss account.

Winter Examination 1998
D Pharm Second Year
Drug Store and Business Management

Q 1. Solve any *five* of the following:

a.   i. Match the following:
   Business means:
   - Trade and commerce
   - Buying and selling of goods
   - Commerce
   - Industry and commerce

    ii. Cash book records _____ transactions only. (Fill in the gap)

b. Enlist the various forms of business organisations.

c. Give objectives of inventory control.

d. Define the term codification of drugs.

e. Define the term cheque. List out the salient features of cheque.

f. Define the following terms:

    i. Assets   iii. Journal

    ii. Liabilities   iv. Ledger

Q 2. Solve any *four* of the following:

a. Give classification of various business activities.

b. Explain the following in short:
   i. Aids to trade   iii. Management
   ii. Commerce

c. Enlist various kinds of partners in the partnership form of business. List out merits and demerits of partnership.

d. Elaborate the channels of distribution in pharmaceutical marketing. Mention various functions of wholesalers.

e. What do you mean by departmental store? Give its merits and demerits.

Q 3. Solve any *four* of the following:

a. Discuss importance of inventory control. What is ABC control of inventory?

b. Define the following terms:
   i. Minimum stock level   iii. Lead time
   ii. Maximum stock level   iv. Safety stock

c. How will you select site of a drug store? What do you mean by layout of a drug store? Give a typical layout of retail drug store.

d. Give common methods of codification of drugs. Give their advantages and disadvantages.

e. Define the term tender. Give important factors in the selection of suppliers.

Q 4. Solve any *four* of the following:

a. Write short notes on:
   i. Economic Order Quantity (EOQ)
   ii. VED analysis

b. Give procedure for scrap and surplus disposal.

c. How is salesmanship important for business? Enlist different qualities a salesman should possess.

d. What factors should be taken into consideration in evaluating the performance of a pharmacist.

e. Write a short account on recruitment and training of pharmacy personnel.

Q 5. Solve any *two* of the following:

a. i. List out kinds of bank accounts. What are the advantages of cash-credit facility.

   ii. Define the term finance. List out the important sources of finance to business.

b. i. Give principles of double entry book-keeping. State its advantages.

ii. Define the term budget. What do you mean by budgetary control?

c. Journalise the following transactions and post them into ledger:

April 1, 1996   Hemraj started business with capital Rs. 51,000

April 10, 1996   He acquired a piece of land for Rs. 20,000

April 25, 1996   Goods worth Rs. 15,000 were purchased from Mr Mohan.

April 25, 1996   Paid to Mr Mohan Rs. 10,000

April 30, 1996   Paid wages Rs. 5,000.

Note—Ignore narration.

Q 6. Solve any *two* of the following:

a. i. What do you understand by the term final statement? Give specimen of profit and loss account.

ii. Why is trial balance is prepared? Discuss the different methods of preparation of trial balance.

b. Give short account on:
   i. Petty cash book
   ii. Financial statements and their analysis

c. Following is the trading and profit and loss account of Navin Medical Store. Prepare balance sheet as on for the year ended March 31, 1995.

Summer Examination 1999
D Pharm Second Year
Drug Store and Business Management

Q 1. Solve any *five* of the following:

a. Define the term 'ledger'.

b. Explain the term 'EOQ'.

c. What is advertising? State its importance.

d. Explain the term "evaluation of a pharmacist".

e. Define the term 'management'.

f. State the objectives of market research.

Q 2. Solve any *four* of the following:

a. What do you understand by 'cash book'? Give its various types.

b. Define salesmanship. What qualities a person should possess to become a successful salesman?

c. State the importance of finance. What are the sources of finance?

d. What is double entry bookkeeping? Explain its principles.

e. Why is pharmaceutical management stated as art and science?

Q 3. Solve any *four* of the following:

a. Give a suitable layout design for wholesale drug store.

b. Define the term 'cheque'. Give types of cheque. Why cheque is crossed at the corner, while making payments to the parties?

c. Explain the term 'turnover rate'. What conclusion can be drawn from low and high turnover?

d. What is re-order level? How it is calculated?

e. Write a format for profit and loss account.

Q 4. Solve any *four* of the following:

a. State any six advantages of budgeting.

b. What is petty cash book? Give a short account. Give its specimen.

c. State the primary functions of medical representative.

d. What is 'Joint Hindu Family' business? Describe its main features.

e. What is 'balance sheet'. Give its format.

Q 5. Solve any *four* of the following:

a. Give a design of a layout of wholesale drug store.

b. Define the terms with suitable examples:
   i. Tender   ii. Contract

c. What are the various sources of finance? Explain the importance of cash-credit facility in developing business.

d. Explain why cash book always shows debit balance.

e. Explain the advantages of window display for retail drug stores.

Q 6. Solve any *four* of the following:

a. Explain the importance of VED analysis technique in inventory control.

b. State the procedures followed in selection of a suitable candidate for salesmanship career.

c. What services we can expect from a bank? Explain the overdraft facility given by the bank.

d. Explain the following concepts:
   i. Inventory carrying cost   ii. Safety stock

e. Define journal. Journalise the following entries for Mr Ram's Account:
   i. 1st March   Received Rs. 3,800 Rent from Mr Patil.
   ii. 2nd March   Paid Rs. 800 to M/s Govind and Sons firm on A/c.

iii. 3rd March Purchased goods worth Rs. 2,500 from
        M/s Decent Agencies on cash payment.

iv. 5th March Sold goods worth Rs. 750 to M/s Decent
        Agencies on credit.

Winter Examination 1999
D Pharm Second Year
Drug Store and Business Management

Q 1. Solve any *five* of the following:

 a. Define the following terms:

   i. Liabilities   iii. Contract

   ii. Industry   iv. Assets

 b. Define the term budgeting. State its importance.

 c. Give objectives of market research.

 d. Define the following terms:

   i. Trial balance   ii. Balance sheet

 e. Define the term 'lead time'.

 f. What do you mean by private enterprises and public enterprises?

 g. State the elements of management.

Q 2. Solve any *four* of the following:

 a. What do you mean by the term management? Explain various functions of management.

 b. Enlist the good qualities of salesman.

 c. Write short note on "window display".

 d. What do you mean by departmental store? Give its merits and demerits.

 e. Define the following terms:

   i. Inventory carrying cost

   ii. Economics

   iii. Cheque

   iv. Compensation

Q 3. Solve any *four* of the following:

 a. Define the term codification of drugs. What are its advantages?

 b. Give the classification of various business activities.

 c. Explain the documents required for the grant of licence for retail drug store.

 d. What do you mean by purchasing? What are its essentials?

 e. Write note on selection of supplier.

Q 4. Solve any *four* of the following:

a. Define the finance. Enlist important sources of finance.

b. What do you mean by salesmanship? Discuss the duties and responsibilities of salesman.

c. Write short account on recruitment and training of pharmacist.

d. Enlist different methods of market research with their merits.

e. Define the term EOQ. Give the importance of inventory control.

Q 5. Solve any *four* of the following:

a. Define the terms:

i. Transaction   iii. Drawings

ii. Debit   iv. Ledger

b. Explain the term profit and loss account and balance sheet.

c. List out kinds of bank account. What are the merits of current account?

d. What do you mean by subsidiary book? Discuss its necessities.

e. Write short note on "bank reconciliation" statement.

Q 6. Solve any *four* of the following:

a. Define the term advertising. Discuss the various media for advertising.

b. Give the objects, importance and utility of book-keeping.

c. What do you mean by:

i. Cash-credit facility   ii. Overdraft facility

d. Define the following terms:

i. Accounting   iii. Trade

ii. Petty cash book

e. Give an example of a typical profit and loss account and balance sheet of the business.

Summer Examination 2000
D Pharm Second Year
Drug Store and Business Management

Q 1. Solve any *five* of the following:

a. Explain the term trade. Enlist various aids to trade.

b. Define the terms:

i. Assets   iii. Gross profit

ii. Transactions   iv. Net profit

c. List different types of partners of partnership form of business.

d. Explain what do you know by evaluation of a pharmacist.

e. Give functions of advertisements. State whether pharmaceuticals are freely advertised.

f. What do you mean by 'tender'? Give its types.

g. What is cash book?

Q 2. Solve any *four* of the following:

a. Enlist different forms of business organisation. Give merits and demerits of partnership.

b. Explain the terms (any *three*):
   i. Business   iii. Industry
   ii. Commerce   iv. Economics

c. What are the advantages of channels of distribution? State the channels of distribution for pharmacy.

d. What do you mean by cooperative form of business? Give its advantages and disadvantages.

e. Write short account on:
   i. Retail departmental store   ii. Multiple shop

Q 3. Solve any *four* of the following:

a. Explain in brief VED analysis and EOQ.

b. What do you understand by the terms:
   i. Lead time   ii. Safety stock

c. Define codification of drugs. State methods of codification. State its advantages.

d. Give objectives of layout. Draw layout design of a drug store.

e. Enlist the legal requirement and different documents required for opening a new drug stores.

Q 4. Solve any *four* of the following:

a. Enlist various sales promotion tools. Write short account on market research.

b. What is salesmanship? Give its importance. Enlist different qualities of salesman.

c. "Window display", one of the forms of advertisement. Explain.

d. Explain the following terms:
   i. Minimum stock level   iii. General ledger
   ii. Maximum stock level

e. Give objectives of inventory control. Enlist different techniques commonly used to control the inventory.

Q 5. Solve any *four* of the following:

a. What do you mean by purchasing? Give its importance. Give objectives of purchasing.

b. Write short account on:
   i. Training of pharmacist
   ii. Statement of profit and loss account.
c. What do you mean by scrap? State procedure for scrap and surplus disposal.
d. What do you know about trial-balance?
e. Explain in brief cash credit and overdraft facility.

Q 6. Solve any *four* of the following:

a. State importance of finance. What are commonly used means in analysing financial statements?
b. Define the term 'budget'. What are the main ôbjectives of budgetary control?
c. What do you mean by double entry book-keeping? State its principle. Give specimen format of:
   i. Journal
   ii. Petty cash book
d. Discuss the objects of preparing "trial balance". Discuss the various errors which are not disclosed by trial balance. Give its format.
e. What are the final accounts? What is the need of preparing a balance sheet? Differentiate between balance sheet and profit and loss account.

Winter Examination 2000
D Pharm Second Year
Drug Store and Business Management

Q 1. Solve any *two* of the following:

a. Which are the legal requirements to start the drug store?
b. State advantages and disadvantages of proprietorship business.
c. How you will generate finance to start the drug store.

Q 2. Solve any *four* of the following:

a. Various display methods in drug store.
b. EOQ model in inventory management.
c. C and F agent and his importance in drug store management.
d. State importance of inventory control. What is lead time?
e. State advantages and disadvantages of partnership form of business.
f. Write short account on:
   i. Bank overdraft facility
   ii. Cash credit facility

Q 3. Solve any *two* of the following:

a. Give typical layout of retail drug store. Enlist various documents required to be submitted for obtaining a retail sale drug licence.

b. Salesmanship and its advantages.

c. Evaluation of a pharmacist and training for a pharmacist.

Q 4. Solve any *two* of the following:

a. Ideal qualities and responsibilities of a good salesman.

b. Advertising methods. Give short account on window display.

c. What is finance? Give sources of finance.

Q 5. Solve any *two* of the following:

a. What do you mean by double entry book-keeping? State its importance.

b. What is trial balance? State its importance. State methods for its preparation.

c. Write short account on balance sheet. Give specimen format of it.

Q 6. Solve any *two* of the following:

a. What do you mean by profit and loss account? Give specimen format of it.

b. Techniques to analyse financial statements.

c. Write short account on cash-credit facility and bank overdraft facility.

Summer Examination 2001
D Pharm Second Year
Drug Store and Business Management

Q 1. Solve any *two* of the following:

a. Factors you will consider to start a new drug store.

b. State advantages and disadvantages of partnership business.

c. Give elements of economics. Define the term trade.

Q 2. Solve any *two* of the following:

a. Which are the various sales promotion methods employed in drug store.

b. Enlist various inventory control techniques. Describe in short ABC and VED analysis.

c. Wholesaler and his importance in drug distribution.

Q 3. Solve any *two* of the following:

a. Wholesaler's supply vs manufacturer's supply.

b. Give layout design of a retail drug store.

c. Enlist the various documents to be submitted to obtain a licence for sale of drugs.

Q 4. Solve any *two* of the following:

a. How will you recruit pharmacist? What do you mean by compensation for a pharmacist?

b. Give services and functions of bank.

c. Give short account of:
    i. Lead time
    ii. Scrap and surplus disposal

Q 5. Solve any *two* of the following:

a. Different kinds of accounts.

b. Define cash book. State its types. What do you mean by petty cash book.

c. Define balance sheet. Give specimen format of it. State its importance.

Q 6. Solve any *two* of the following:

a. Which are the objectives of bookkeeping? Give advantages and disadvantages of double entry bookkeeping.

b. Give short account of profit and loss account.

c. Importance of budgetary. What do you mean by budgetary control?

Winter Examination 2001
D Pharm Second Year
Drug Store and Business Management

Q 1. Solve any *five* of the following:

a. Define the term aids to trade. Enlist various aids to trade.

b. What do you mean by "petty cash book"?

c. Define partnership. Enlist merits and demerits of partnership form of business.

d. Define the following terms:
    i. Business   iii. Commerce
    ii. Lead time   iv. Assets

e. Name the different channels of distribution of drugs.

f. State different types of bank accounts.

g. Give the objectives of inventory control.

Q 2. Solve any *four* of the following:

a. What do you mean by codification of drugs? Enlist various types of codification and merits.

b. Discuss various forms of business organisation in short.

c. Enlist the elements of economics.

d. What do you mean by tender? Explain various types of tenders.

e. Define the following terms:

    i. Minimum stock level.   iii. VED analysis

    ii. Maximum stock level.   iv. Safety stock

Q 3. Solve any *four* of the following:

a. What do you mean by layout of drug store? How will you select the site of drug store?

b. Define purchasing. Enlist objectives of purchasing.

c. What is 'ABC' techniques of inventory control?

d. What are factors to be taken into consideration for the selection of supplier?

e. Write short note on 'bank cash credit facility'.

Q 4. Solve any *four* of the following:

a. Define 'salesmanship'. Explain the qualities of salesman.

b. Explain the purchase procedure in detail for pharmaceutical products.

c. What do you mean by EOQ (Economic Order Quantity)? How does it help to maintain safety stock?

d. Define the marketing. Explain the functions of marketing.

e. Explain the procedure to be followed for the disposal of surplus stock.

Q 5. Solve any *four* of the following:

a. Define the terms:

    i. Account   iii. Journal

    ii. Overdraft   iv. Credit

b. Enlist different sources of finance.

c. What do you mean by ledger? Give specimen format of it.

d. Define bookkeeping. What are the merits of double entry book-keeping?

e. Discuss the different methods of preparation of trial balance.

Q 6. Solve any *four* of the following:

a. What is master budget? What are the requirements for an effective budgetary control.

b. Define the following terms:

    i. Debenture

    ii. Trial balance

    iii. Codification of drug

c. Enlist various types of bank accounts. Give salient features of cheque.

d. Define cash book. Enlist types of cash book. Give its objectives.

e. What is balance sheet? Give proforma of:

    i. Balance sheet   ii. Profit and loss account

Summer Examination 2002
D Pharm Second Year
Drug Store and Business Management

Q 1. Solve any *five* of the following:

a. Give the objectives of inventory control.

b. Define the term "economics".

c. State the rules of making entries in the cash book.

d. What do you mean by "lead time"?

e. Define the term codification of drugs.

f. Define the following terms (any *two*)

    i. Solvency

    ii. Ledger

    iii. Recruitment

    iv. Cheque

Q 2. Solve any *four* of the following:

a. Define management. What are the advantages and disadvantages of cooperative business organisation.

b. Explain the terms:

    i. Trade

    ii. Commerce

    iii. Aids to trade

c. How will you select a site for retail medical stores to be located in a town?

d. How is disposal of surplus stock carried out?

e. Define sales promotion. What are objectives of sales promotion?

Q 3. Solve any *four* of the following:

a. State the functions of departmental stores. Give the demerits of departmental stores.

b. Define the term 'bank'. State any three fundamental functions carried out by the bank.

c. Define purchasing. State objectives of purchasing.

d. State the qualities and duties of medical representative.

e. State the functions of drug wholesaler.

Q 4. Solve any *four* of the following:

a. What are advertising? Which method of advertising is suitable for promotion of ethical products?

b. State objectives of inventory control. Write short account on VED analysis.

c. Explain the terms (any *two*):
   i. Acid test ratio
   ii. Current ratio
   iii. Net working capital turnover
   iv. Ratio analysis

d. What is 'trial balance' statement? Give specimen format of it.

e. State the management functions which are fulfilled through market research (Any *six* functions).

Q 5. Solve any *four* of the following:

a. State the types of accounts. How will you journalise the following entries for Mr Ram's account?
   i. 1st March   Received Rs. 3,500/- loan from Dena bank
   ii. 3rd March   Purchased table and chairs worth Rs. 2,000/- from M/s Modern Furnitures on cash payment.
   iii. 7th March   Paid house rent Rs. 1,000/- to Mr Desai.
   iv. 8th March   Sold goods worth Rs. 950/- to Mr Ashok on credit.

b. How prices of drugs are determined? State formula of calculation of retail price of a formulation.

c. Define the terms (any *two*):
   i. Journal
   ii. Cash book
   iii. Petty cash book

d. What is ABC analysis? Describe its importance.

e. What is training? Give its types. State the various aspects to be covered during training of a salesman.

Q 6. Solve any *four* of the following:

a. Explain the concept of budget. State the advantages of budgetary control method.

b. Give the specimen format for the balance sheet.

c. State the importance of finance. Give various sources of finance.

d. What legal requirements are to be fulfilled to start a retail drug store?

e. Explain pharmaceutical marketing process with the help of a suitable chart.

Winter Examination 2002
D Pharm Second Year
Drug Store and Business Management

Q 1. Solve any *five* of the following:

    a. Define the following terms:

        i. Management   iii. Budget

        ii. Journal   iv. Contract

    b. What do you mean by lead time?

    c. Explain the term 'EOQ'.

    d. State the objective of market research.

    e. What are the different kinds of accounts?

    f. Give the qualities of successful salesman.

    g. Explain why training of pharmacist is necessary.

Q 2. Solve any *four* of the following:

    a. Define the terms with examples:

        i. Tender   ii. Codification

    b. What is partnership? Explain the merits and demerits of partnership form of business organisation.

    c. Define 'industry'. Classify and explain in detail 'manufacturing industry'.

    d. Explain wholesaler and his importance in drug distribution.

    e. Discuss the legal requirements and different documents required for opening a new drug store.

Q 3. Solve any *four* of the following:

    a. Explain the following concepts:

        i. Inventory carrying cost   iii. Surplus

        ii. Safety stock

    b. What is sales promotion? Describe objectives of sales promotion.

    c. Explain window display is one of the forms of advertisement.

    d. Define 'inventory control'. Discuss the objectives and importance of inventory control.

    e. What do you mean by scrap? State the procedure for scrap and surplus disposal.

Q 4. Solve any *four* of the following:

    a. Define the following terms:

        i. Economics   iii. Retailer

        ii. Commerce   iv. Partnership deed

    b. What is 'Joint Hindu Family' business? Describe its main features.

c. Define 'financial statement'. Enlist different methods used for financial analysis.

d. What do you mean by compensation for a pharmacist? Write short account on recruitment of a pharmacist.

e. Write a short account on:
    i. Sole proprietorship   ii. Multiple shop

Q 5. Solve any *four* of the following:

a. Define the following terms:
    i. Cash book
    ii. Drawing
    iii. Cheque
    iv. VED analysis

b. Give services and functions of bank.

c. Define 'accounting'. Enlist the main objectives of accounting.

d. What do you mean by 'petty cash book'? State its principle and give specimen format.

e. Define 'trial balance'. State the errors that occur in trial balance. Discuss any one method of preparing trial balance.

Q 6. Solve any *four* of the following:

a. Define the following terms:
    i. Debenture
    ii. Liability
    iii. Overdraft
    iv. Bad debts

b. What do you mean by 'budgetary control'? Discuss its advantages.

c. Write a short account on 'fixed capital' and 'working capital'.

d. What is the object of preparing profit and loss account? Give proforma of profit and loss account.

e. Journalise the following entries for Amit Medical Store's Account.

Year 2002	Particulars	Rs.
1st June	Purchase goods for cash	15,000/-
5th June	Paid salaries	3,000/-
6th June	Sold goods for cash	20,000/-
12th June	Purchase furniture from M/s-X	3,000/-
14th June	Received from Mr Shubham	900/-
16th June	Paid to Mrs Sheetal Jaiswal	11,200/-
20th June	Received commission	500/-

Summer Examination 2003
D Pharm Second Year
Drug Store and Business Management

Q 1. Attempt the following:

a. Define the terms (any *two*)
   i. Trade   iii. Business
   ii. Economics

b. State the disadvantages of the sole proprietorship business.

c. Name the different channels for distribution of drugs.

d. Define 'mail order business'. State the main types of mail order business.

e. State the minimum qualifications required to start retail drug store and wholesale drug store.

f. State the objectives of trial balance statement.

g. What are the advantages of codification of drugs in drug stores?

Q 2. Solve any *four* of the following:

a. Give classification of budget.

b. Describe the advantages and limitations of financial statements.

c. What is the difference between journal and ledger?

d. State the advantages and disadvantages of partnership form of business.

e. Describe in short the steps involved in selling process used in sale of drugs.

Q 3. Solve any *four* of the following:

a. State the advantages of the perpetual inventory system.

b. State the advantages and disadvantages of 'Joint Hindu Family' form of business.

c. State the functions of the wholesalers.

d. What is the difference between departmental stores and multiple shops?

e. How is profit and loss account prepared?

Q 4. Solve any *four* of the following:

a. Write a note on 'window display' arranged in drug stores.

b. State the difference between over-draft facility and cash-credit facility of a commercial bank.

c. Explain the entity concept and dual aspect concept used in accountancy.

d. Mention the main books of original entry used in recording business transactions. Give the format of cash book.

e. How are profitability ratio calculated by using various methods?

Q 5. Solve any *four* of the following:

a. Give typical layout of retail drug store. Enlist various documents required to be submitted for obtaining a retail sale drug licence.

b. State the ideal qualities and responsibilities of a good salesman.

c. Define the following terms:
   i. VED analysis   iii. Purchases journal
   ii. Capital turnover ratio

d. State the main functions of the budget committee.

e. State the items included in balance sheet.

Q 6. Solve any *four* of the following:

a. Define 'scrap'. Give its classification. How is scrap controlled in pharmaceutical manufacturing company?

b. State the factors to be taken into consideration while selecting a supplier.

c. How is evaluation of the pharmacist carried out?

d. Describe the various aspects to be covered during market research.

e. Define 'tender'. Write a note on any 3 types of tender.

Winter Examination 2003
D Pharm Second Year
Drug Store and Business Management

Q 1. Solve any *five* of the following:

a. Define the terms (any *two*):
   i. Commerce   iii. Industry
   ii. Management

b. Why is storage of goods necessary?

c. What services are given by the retailer to manufacturer and wholesaler?

d. Define "distribution channels."

e. Specify the minimum desirable areas to open new retail drug stores and new wholesale drug stores.

f. Mention the types of errors which are not reflected in trial balance statement.

g. What steps are taken to detect slow and nonmoving items in the stores?

Q 2. Solve any *four* of the following:

a. State the importance of inventory control. What is lead time?

b. State the advantages and disadvantages of 'consumer cooperative stores form of business.

c. State the various points to be taken into consideration while purchasing the materials.

d. How is pricing of materials calculated by using FIFO and LIFO methods?

e. State the limitations of budgetary control method.

Q 3. Solve any *four* of the following:

a. Describe ABC analysis technique used to control inventroy.

b. State the advantages of 'joint stock company' form of business.

c. Describe the functions of the retailers.

d. Write a note on 'Economic Ordering Quantity (EOQ)'.

e. How is finance raised for starting a new drug store?

Q 4. Solve any *four* of the following:

a. Describe in brief the various techniques used in sales promotion.

b. Give layout design for retail drug stores.

c. Define 'accounting convention'. Explain any *two* conventions commonly used in preparation of accounting statements.

d. Give classification of accounts used in double entry bookkeeping system.

e. How is financial analysis carried out? Explain by using any *two* methods.

Q 5. Solve any *four* of the following:

a. What is trial balance? State the method for preparation of trial balance.

b. Define 'marketing'. Explain functions of marketing.

c. What is the importance of profit and loss account? Give the specimen format of profit and loss account.

d. Define the following terms:
   i. Inventory turnover ratio
   ii. Net profit ratio
   iii. Budget

e. State the essential features of good advertisement.

Q 6. Solve any *four* of the following:

a. Write a note on petty cash book. Give its format.

b. How minimum stock level and re-order level is fixed to maintain inventory control?

c. Specify the various points to be included in the training programme planned for the pharmacists.
d. State the advantages of market research.
e. Enlist different types of partners under partnership form of business.

Summer Examination 2004
D Pharm Second Year
Drug Store and Business Management

Q 1. Attempt any *five* of the following:
a. Define the following terms:
    i. Business   iii. Salesmanship
    ii. Bank   iv. Finance
b. What do you mean by 'ledger'?
c. Explain the term 'evaluation of pharmacist'.
d. State the objectives of layout design of drug store.
e. What is advertising? State its importance.
f. Explain the types of discount.
g. Give the functions of management.

Q 2. Solve any *four* of the following:
a. Define the following terms with examples:
    i. Purchasing
    ii. Contracts
b. What is layout of drug store? Give design of layout of a retail drug store.
c. Discuss various kinds of partners in a partnership of business.
d. Define the term 'trade'. Enlist aids to trade. Give elements of economics.
e. What are the advantages of channels of distribution? State the channels of distribution of pharmacy.

Q 3. Solve any *four* of the following:
a. What do you know about minimum and maximum stock level?
b. Explain the importance of VED analysis technique in inventory control.
c. State the primary functions of medical representative.
d. What do you mean by market research? Give its advantages.
e. The annual consumption of a material is 700 units, the cost of material is Rs. 50/- per unit and ordering cost is Rs. 43/- per unit.
    The storage and carrying cost is 12% of inventory control.
    Find out the EOQ and number of orders to be placed per year.

Q 4. Solve any *four* of the following:

a. Define the following terms:
  i. Assets iii. Gross profit
  ii. Transactions iv. Net profit

b. What do you mean by multiple shop? Explain the features of mail order business.

c. Why pharmaceutical management is stated an art and science?

d. What are sources of finance? State the importance of finances.

e. Write a short account on:
  i. Cooperative societies
  ii. Foreign trade

Q 5. Solve any *four* of the following:

a. Define the following terms:
  i. Account iii. Book-keeping
  ii. Capital iv. Crossed cheque

b. What do you mean by bearer and order cheque? Why are cheques crossed at the corner, while making payments to the parties?

c. Explain in brief cash credit and overdraft facility.

d. State the object of preparing trial balance. Give its format.

e. Discuss in detail double entry book-keeping system.

Q 6. Solve any *four* of the following:

a. Explain the following terms:
  i. Codification of drug
  ii. Bill of exchange

b. Define the term 'budget'. Discuss the objectives of budgetary control.

c. What is the need of preparing a balance sheet? Give a proforma of balance sheet.

d. Write short account on:
  i. Purchase book
  ii. Financial planning

e. Journalise the following entries in simple cash book of M/s Amit Traders for the month of June 2002.
  i. Borrowed Rs. 10,000/- from bank and introduced capital Rs. 8,000/-.
  ii. Paid salary Rs. 3,000/- and wages Rs. 550/-.
  iii. Cash purchases Rs. 6,000/- at 10% TD.
  iv. Paid life insurance premium of Rs. 750/- and fire insurance of Rs. 1,000/-.
  v. Cash sales of Rs. 8,000/- at 5% TD.

Winter Examination 2004
D Pharm Second Year
Drug Store and Business Management

Q 1. Solve any *five* of the following:

a. Define the terms (any *two*):
      i. Accounting   iii. Bank
      ii. Business

b. Explain 'ledger'.

c. Explain the types of discount.

d. Give the objectives of inventory control.

e. Define 'retailer'. What are their functions?

f. What are the limitations of budgetary control?

g. Explain the term 'EOQ'.

Q 2. Solve any *four* of the following:

a. What is 'trade'? Give classification of trade.

b. Describe a well-organised selection procedure for selection of a pharmacist.

c. What is 'financial planning'? Give various types of finance.

d. Define 'industry'. Explain various types of manufacturing industries.

e. Define 'tender'. Explain various types of tenders.

Q 3. Solve any *four* of the following:

a. Explain 'perpetual inventory system'. Give its advantages.

b. What is a cash book? Describe various types of cash books.

c. List various methods of financial analysis.

d. What are the advantages of 'codification of drugs' in a drug store? Give various methods of codification.

e. Write in detail about 'mail order business'.

Q 4. Solve any *four* of the following:

a. What is 'profit and loss account'? Give format of:
      i. Profit and loss account   ii. Balance sheet

b. Differentiate between a 'departmental store' and multiple shops.

c. Give a typical layout of a retail drug store. Mention various documents required to be submitted for getting a retail drug store licence.

d. What is 'sales promotion'? Describe various techniques of sales promotion.

e. What are 'accounting concept'? Explain 'money measurement concept' and 'dual aspect concept' used in accountacy.

Q 5. Solve any *four* of the following:

a. Explain the following terms (any *two*):
   i. Drawing
   ii. Overdraft
   iii. Debenture
   iv. Petty cash book

b. What is 'trial balance'? Write various objectives and any one method of preparation of the trial balance.

c. Define' budgetary control'. Give classification of budgets.

d. Explain about various types of middlemen in the trade.

e. Define 'partnership'. State various kinds of partners.

Q 6. Solve any *four* of the following:

a. What are the various steps involved in purchasing procedure?

b. Write in details about 'accounting errors'.

c. Discuss the advantages and disadvantages of cooperative business organisation.

d. Explain, window display as an effective form of advertisement.

e. Enlist various inventory control techniques. Describe in short VED analysis.

Summer Examination 2005
D Pharm Second Year
Drug Store and Business Management

Q 1. Answer any *five* of the following:

a. Define the term 'aids to trade'. Name important aids to trade.

b. Write short note on 'elements of economics'.

c. i. Define the terms 'commerce' and 'management'.
   ii. What do you understand by pharmaceutical management?

d. What do you understand by:
   i. Tender
   ii. Contract

e. Discuss the limitations of 'Economic Ordering Quantity (EOQ)'.

f. Define the following terms:
   i. Assets
   ii. Liabilities
   iii. Transaction
   iv. Credit

g. Define the following terms:
   i. Trial balance
   ii. Balance sheet

Q 2. Answer any *four* of the following:

a. Give the advantages and disadvantages of 'cooperative business organisation'.

b. Enlist various kinds of partners in the partnership form of business. Give the merits and demerits of partnership.

c. What is 'Joint Hindu Family business'? Describe its main features.

d. Discuss the importance and objectives of inventory control.

e. Mention different methods of inventory control. Give advantages of perpetual inventory control system.

f.   i. Explain the terms 'minimum' and maximum' level of inventory.

   ii. What is Re-Order Level (ROL)?

Q 3. Answer any *four* of the following:

a. What are the factors to be considered for the selection of suppliers?

b. What do you understand by 'market research'? Explain its objectives.

c. "Window display is one of the forms of advertisement." Explain.

d. What factors should be taken into consideration in evaluating the performance of a pharmacist?

e. Give a short account of 'recruitment and training of pharmacist'.

f. Define 'salesmanship. What qualities a person should possess to become successful salesman?

Q 4. Answer any *four* of the following:

a. How will you select site for a drug store? What do you mean by layout of drug store?

b. What are the legal requirements and general conditions for opening a drug store?

c. Give a typical layout of a drug store.

d. Give common methods of codification of drugs. Give their advantages and disadvantages.

e. What do you mean by departmental store? Give its merits and demerits.

f. Give a short account of "multiple shop".

Q 5. Answer any *four* of the following:

a. Define the term finance. Give the important sources of finance to business.

b. What services can we expect from a bank? Explain the overdraft facility given by the bank.

c. List out kinds of bank accounts. What are the advantages of current account?

d. What do you mean by double entry bookkeeping? Explain its principles.

e. What do you understand by 'cash book'? Give its various types.

f. What do you mean by subsidiary books? Discuss its necessities.

Q 6. Answer any *four* of the following:

a. Explain the term 'general ledger'. Distinguish between 'journal' and 'ledger'.

b. Discuss different methods of preparation of 'trial balance'. State various errors which are not disclosed by the trial balance.

c. Write a short note on 'bank reconciliation statement'.

d. What is the need of preparing a balance sheet? Differentiate between 'balance sheet' and 'profit and loss account'.

e. i. Define 'financial analysis'.

    ii. What are the different methods used for financial analysis?

f. Define the term 'budgeting'. State its importance.

Winter Examination 2005
D Pharm Second Year
Drug Store and Business Management

Q 1. Solve any *five* of the following:

a. Define the terms:

    i. Pharmaceutical management ii. Contract

b. State the disadvantages of 'joint stock company' form of business.

c. Define 'tender' and mention different types of tenders.

d. State the different tests that are commonly used in the election procedure of a 'pharmacist'.

e. Define the term 'goods' and give the four categories in which goods account is divided.

f. What is contra entry? How is it distinguished in the cash book from other entries?

g. Define the term 'bank' and mention different types of banks.

Q 2. Solve any *four* of the following:

a. Define the term "trade". Give its classification.

b. Describe the salient features of "Joint Hindu Family" business.

c. Differentiate between wholesalers and retailers.

d. Explain the term 'perpetual inventory system' and mention main advantages.

e. Explain the three objectives of budgetary control.

Q 3. Solve any *four* of the following:

a. Explain the term 'industry' and give its classification on the basis of size and investment.

b. Discuss the general factors to be considered while selecting a site for a drug store.

c. Discuss the advantages of 'advertising'.

d. What is double entry bookkeeping? Give the advantages of double entry bookkeeping.

e. Differentiate between 'profit and loss account' and 'balance sheet'.

Q 4. Solve any *four* of the following:

a. What are the advantages of 'sole proprietorship business'?

b. Define the term 'purchase procedure' and explain the various stages of purchase procedure.

c. What is meant by 'market research'? Write about the various methods of market research.

d. What is meant by the term 'financial planning'? Mention main aspects of financial planning.

e. Give the requirements of effective budgeting.

Q 5. Solve any *four* of the following:

a. Describe the main advantages of 'multiple shops'.

b. Define the term 'inventory' and state the various functions of inventory control.

c. Discuss the various plans of compensating an efficient pharmacist to maintain the interest in his job.

d. Describe the terms:
   i. Fixed capital
   ii. Working capital
   iii. Loan capital

e. Prepare a simple cash book from the following transactions of Mr Ravi of M/s Getwell Pharmacy for the month of December, 2003.

Year 2003	Particulars	Rs.
December 1	Mr Ravi started business with cash	85,000/-
December 4	Purchased goods for cash	4,000/-
December 5	Sold goods for cash	4,350/-
December 6	Bought furniture for cash	2,700/-
December 7	Received commission	200/-
December 8	Purchased goods from Shyamlal and paid cash	2,100/-
December 9	Withdraw cash for personal use	4,000/-
December 10	Paid salaries	4,450/-

Q 6. Solve any *four* of the following:

a. Mention the important features of 'hire purchase trading house'.

b. Explain the terms:
   i. Maximum stock level
   ii. Minimum stock level
   iii. Recorder level
   iv. Danger level

c. Define the term 'sales promotion'. Mention the objectives of sales promotion.

d. Describe 'compensating errors' and 'errors of omission with suitable examples.

e. Define the following terms:
   i. Debt-equity ratio
   ii. Current ratio
   iii. Gross profit ratio

Summer Examination 2006
D Pharm Second Year
Drug Store and Business Management

Q 1. Answer any *five* of the following:

a. Define trade. Which are the various trades covered under foreign trade.

b. What do you mean by 'partnership deed'? Name the various types of partners.

c. Define wholesaler. Classify the different types of wholesaler.

d. Write the formula to calculate the retail price of a drug formulation.

e. Write the classification of scrap along with its method for disposal.

f. State the advantages of window display.

g. What is the difference between overdraft and cash credit.

Q 2. Answer any *four* of the following:

a. Define finance. What do you mean by the word 'long-term finance'.

b. Which are the various methods of market research? What are advantages and disadvantages of telephone interview method?

c. What are A, B, C types of inventories? Write the advantages of ABC analysis.

d. Write the various documents needed to open a new retail drug store.

e. Mention the salient features of hire purchase trading house along with its advantages and disadvantages.

f. State the difference between sole proprietorship and partnership.

Q 3. Answer any *four* of the following:

   a. What are the various functions of management?

   b. What is 'Joint Hindu Family' business? Write its salient features.

   c. Define retailer. Give the various functions of retailer and the services rendered to producer or wholesaler by him.

   d. Give the various steps of purchase procedure.

   e. What is EOQ? Give the various methods of finding EOQ.

   f. Define 'salesman'. What are the different qualities of good salesman.

Q 4. Answer any *four* of the following:

   a. Define 'selection'. What are the steps involved in selection procedure?

   b. What are commercial banks? Give the various functions and services offered by commercial bank.

   c. What does perpetual inventory system comprise of? Give the format for a bin card.

   d. Define 'codification'. Write the different methods of codification.

   e. What is cooperative society? Give the main features of it.

   f. What is called consumer goods and producers goods? Write classification of industry based on size and investment.

Q 5. Answer any *four* of the following:

   a. Write the various activities revolving around trade.

   b. Give a typical layout of a drug store.

   c. Define 'tender'. What are different types of tender.

   d. What is VED analysis?

   e. What are the objectives of advertising? Which different media are used for advertisement?

   f. How is the recruitment of a pharmacist done?

Q 6. Answer any *four* of the following:

   a. Define the following terms:

       i. Asset   iii. Ledger

       ii. Transaction   iv. Bad debt

   b. What is a difference between journal and ledger?

   c. What are different types of accounts along with their debit credit.

   d. Define trial balance. What are the objectives of the trial balance?

   e. What is financial statement? What information do they provide? State the advantages of it?

   f. What are the main books of original entry? Give the format for journal.

Winter Examination 2006
D Pharm Second Year
Drug Store and Business Management

Q 1. Answer any *five* of the following:

a. Write in brief the functions of the bank.

b. What do you know about minimum and maximum stock levels?

c. Discuss the salient features of the master budget.

d. Define the following terms:
 i. Economic order quantity iii. Capital
 ii. Commerce iv. Turnover

e. Define the term tender. Discuss different types of tenders.

f. State various sources of the finance.

g. Discuss mail order business in brief.

Q 2. Answer any *four* of the following:

a. State the functions of the management.

b. Define aids to trade. Discuss different aids to trade.

c. Write the functions of the wholesaler.

d. Discuss the factors affecting selection of site for drug store.

e. State importance and objectives of purchasing.

Q 3. Answer any *four* of the following:

a. Discuss methods of drug codification with its merits and demerits.

b. Define cooperative business. State its advantages and disadvantages.

c. State factors affecting the selection of suppliers.

d. State minimum legal requirements to start the drug store.

e. State qualities of good salesman.

Q 4. Answer any *four* of the following:

a. State importance of window display in pharmaceutical sale.

b. Discuss the procedure for disposal of scrap and surplus.

c. State importance of market research with its advantages and disadvantages.

d. Discuss ABC analysis of inventory control.

e. What do you know about lead time. Explain in brief.

Q 5. Answer any *four* of the following:

a. State the methods of evaluation of performance of the pharmacist.

b. Differentiate between partnership and joint stock company business.

c. State the methods of preparation of trial balance.

d. State objectives of bookkeeping.

e. Draw a specimen format of petty cash book.

Q 6. Answer any *four* of the following:

a. Explain the methods of compensation to the pharmacist.

b. What is accounting concept? Explain "going concern and money measurement concept" of accountancy.

c. Explain in brief methods of analyzing the financial statements.

d. State how will you prepare the profit and loss account and balance sheet.

e. Explain the following terms (any *two*):
   i. Bad debts   iii. Debenture
   ii. General ledger

Summer Examination 2007
D Pharm Second Year
Drug Store and Business Management

Q 1. Answer any *five* of the following:

a. Mention four functional areas of management.

b. Mention any four services of a wholesaler to a manufacturer.

c. Give formula for economic ordering quantity (EOQ) and mention assumptions in the calculation of EOQ.

d. Mention any four factors for selection of a site for a drug store.

e. Define balance sheet (BS) and give its format.

f. Give equation of trading account.

g. Mention the purpose of preparation of final accounts. What does it consist of?

Q 2. Answer any *four* of the following:

a. Define aids to trade. List its auxiliaries. Explain in brief how transportation helps trade.

b. Define "tender". Explain different types of tenders.

c. Write three merits of each partnership and Joint Hindu Family (JHF) business.

d. Discuss the advantages and disadvantages of joint stock company.

e. What is VED analysis?

f. What is double entry bookkeeping? Give rules of debit and credit to personal, real and nominal accounts.

Q 3. Answer any *four* of the following:

a. Give meaning of distribution. Mention methods of selling adopted by a producer of pharmaceutical products.

b. Mention objectives of an ideal layout design for a drug store and draw typical layout of it.

    c. Define inventory. Mention objectives and functions of inventory control.

    d. Give meaning of market. Classify market.

    e. Define the following:

       i. Recruitment   iii. Induction

       ii. Selection   iv. Training

    f. Define bank. Give kinds of banks. Mention functions of commercial banks.

Q 4. Answer any *four* of the following:

    a. Define cheque. Mention its types. Draw the typical cheque with its contents.

    b. Give types of financial needs of a business. Explain fixed capital and working capital.

    c. Give meaning of budget and budgetary control. Mention advantages of budgetary control.

    d. Mention techniques of financial analysis. Give advantages of ratio analysis.

    e. Give meaning of business organization (BO). Classify ownership forms of BO. Mention four important factors according to you that help in choosing a BO suitable for starting a drug store in a locality.

    f. Define purchasing. Mention its objectives. Write in brief about importance of purchasing to a businessman.

Q 5. Answer any *four* of the following:

    a. Mention features of departmental form of organization. Give its merits and demerits.

    b. Differentiate between a retailer and wholesaler on following points:

       i. Location

      ii. Window display

     iii. Scale of operation

     iv. Nature of business

      v. Profit margin

     vi. Specialization

    vii. Clientage

    c. Give a short account of multiple shop.

    d. Give importance of sales promotion in view of manufacturers, middlemen, consumer.

    e. Define book-keeping and accountancy. What does accounting cycle include? Mention four main objectives of book-keeping and acountancy.

    f. Give long form of 'GAAP'. Mention any three accounting concepts and any three accounting conventions.

Q 6. Answer any *four* of the following:

a. Analyse the transactions in seven steps, "Commenced business with cash Rs. 15,000".

b. Mention different "source documents". Draw a typical 'cash memo' for National Medical and General Stores, New Delhi.

Source documents: Vouchers, invoices, bills, cash memos, receipts.

c. Journalize the following transactions in the journal of National Medical and General Stores, New Delhi.

01-06-2005	Ranjan invested in business	Rs. 20,000
02-06-2005	Open an account with SBI by depositing cash	Rs. 10,000
03-06-2005	Purchased goods for cash	Rs. 500
04-06-2005	Withdrawn cash for personal use	Rs. 200
05-06-2005	Cash sales	Rs. 900
26-06-2005	Paid rent	Rs. 125
30-06-2005	Paid cartage	Rs. 110

d. Define management. Mention features of management. Mention four functions of management.

e. Define partnership deed. List 6 most important contents of partnership deed. Give limitations of an unregistered partnership deed.

f. Define business. Mention any *two* essential features of business. Mention four objectives of busi.:ess.

Summer Examination 2008
D Pharm Second Year
Drug Store and Business Management

Q 1. Answer any *five* of the following:

a. State different types of bank accounts.

b. Define the term partnership. Give the merits of partnership.

c. What is 'safety stock' and 'inventory carrying cost'?

d. State the objectives of market research.

e. What do you mean by 'tender'? Give its types.

f. Give the salient features of retailers.

g. Define the following terms:
  i. Recruitment
  ii. Training
  iii. Placement
  iv. Selection

Q 2. Answer any *four* of the following:

a. What do you mean by the term 'purchasing? Describe importance and objectives of purchasing.
b. Define the term 'codification'. Discuss advantages of codification.
c. Discuss the factors which should be considered for the selection of site of a retail drug store.
d. Give the advantages and disadvantages of opening a drug store in a rural or small town.
e. Define salesman. Give the qualities of successful salesman.
f. Define 'sales promotion'. Describe various sources of market research.

Q 3. Answer any *four* of the following:

a. Give classification of various business activities.
b. Explain various hindrances which arise in trade and discuss how these hindrances can be removed.
c. Differentiate between a 'firm' and a 'company'.
d. Describe the salient features of a cooperative society business.
e. Explain the procedure to be followed for scrap and surplus disposal.
f. What do you understand by the term 'inventory'? Describe objectives and importance of inventory control.

Q 4. Answer any *four* of the following:

a. Discuss the functions of a wholesaler.
b. Give the advantages and disadvantages of 'mail order business'.
c. Define the term 'middlemen'. Enumerate briefly various types of middlemen and explain merchantile agents in detail.
d. Why is training of pharmacists necessary? Discuss how the services rendered by a pharmacist can be compensated.
e. Describe short-term and medium-term financial sources.
f. What do you mean by a bank? Explain the functions of a bank.

Q 5. Answer any *four* of the following:

a. Give the objectives of book-keeping. Explain the principles of double entry book-keeping.
b. Define the following terms:
  i. Debit
  ii. Capital
  iii. Goods
  iv. Insolvent
c. Define the term 'accounting'. Enumerate various 'accounting concepts' and 'accounting conventions'.

d. Define the term 'trial balance'. What are the advantages of preparing trial balance?

e. If the debit side and credit side of a trial balance agree in amount, is this a conclusive proof of the accuracy of ledger accounts? If not, what are the errors which remain undetected in the trial balance?

f. i. What is ledger? Why is it called the principal book of accounts?

ii. Define 'journal' and 'cash book'.

Q 6. Answer any *four* of the following:

a. From the following transactions, make journal entries and post them in ledger.

March 31 rent Rs. 800, Wages Rs. 500 and Salaries Rs. 1,200 paid in cash.

b. Differentiate between 'profit and loss account' and 'balance sheet'.

c. What do you understand by 'petty cash book'? Give a specimen format of 'petty cash book'.

d. Explain in brief the different methods of 'financial analysis'.

e. How will you include the following items while preparing a profit and loss account?

i. Salaries   v. Income-tax

ii. Discount   vi. Advertisement

iii. Commission   vii. Bad debts

iv. Repairs

f. i. What are the different basis for classification of budget?

ii. Give two advantages of budgetary control.

iii. Give two limitations of budgetary control.

Summer Examination 2009
D Pharm Second Year
Drug Store and Business Management

Q 1. Answer any *five* of the following:

a. Define the following terms:

i. Tender   iii. Commerce

ii. Lead time   iv. Capital

b. State different types of bank account.

c. Give objectives of inventory control.

d. What are the advantages of drug codification in drug stores?

e. Give the functions of management.

f. Give the qualities of a good salesman.

g. State the method for preparation of trial balance.

Q 2. Answer any *four* of the following:

a. Give the advantages and disadvantages of joint stock company business.

b. Describe in short ABC analysis.

c. State what do you know about safety stock?

d. Write in brief about EOQ.

e. Define wholesaler. Write his importance in drug distribution.

f. State the types of partners.

Q 3. Answer any *four* of the following:

a. Define purchasing. State objectives of purchasing.

b. What legal requirements are to be fulfilled to start a retail drug store?

c. State factors affecting the selection of suppliers.

d. Give ideal layout design of a retail drug store.

e. Define aids to trade. State different aids to trade.

f. State elements of economics.

Q 4. Answer any *four* of the following:

a. "Window display is a silent salesman". Explain.

b. Give services and functions of the bank.

c. What do you understand by 'market research'? Write advantages and disadvantages of market research.

d. State different modes of sales promotion in drug store.

e. State the functions of retailers.

f. Define advertisement. State its importance.

Q 5. Answer any *four* of the following:

a. State how will you design the training programme for pharmacist working in drug store?

b. Explain in brief 'separate entity' and 'dual aspect' concepts used in accountancy.

c. Write short account on balance sheet. Give specimen format of it.

d. State how profit and loss account is prepared?

e. Define the term 'budgeting'. State its importance.

f. State how evaluation of the pharmacist is carried out.

Q 6. Answer any *four* of the following:

a. Define bookkeeping. Write objectives of double entry system of bookkeeping.

b. How is financial analysis carried out? Explain by using any one method.

c. Write the sources of finance.

d. What do you know about 'petty cash book'? Give its speciman format.

e. State the procedure for scrap and surplus disposal.

f. Journalise the following transactions in Suresh Medical Store Account.

Year 2004	Particulars	Rs.
1 January	Purchased goods for cash	10,000
4 January	Purchased furniture	500
8 January	Sold goods for cash	2,000
15 January	Received from Ramesh	700
18 January	Sold goods to Rajesh	400
20 January	Paid salaries	200
25 January	Received commission	100

Summer Examination 2010
D Pharm Second Year
Drug Store and Business Management

Q 1. Answer any *ten* of the following:

a. Define the terms (any *two*):
   i. Commerce
   ii. Trade
   iii. Contract

b. Define 'Industry'. Write the types of manufacturing industry.

c. State the qualities of good salesman.

d. Explain in brief safety stock level.

e. State the advantages of window display.

f. Define 'Aids to trade'. Enlist various aids to trade.

g. Write main features of joint Hindu family business.

h. State the difference between Private and Public Limited Company.

i. State the functions of the management.

j. Define 'Tender'. List different types of tenders.

k. Explain in brief the 'Lead Time'.

l. Write utility functions of the bank.

m. Define codification. Enlist its methods.

n. Write methods of preparation of trial balance.

Q 2. Answer any *three* of the following:

a. Define 'Partnership'. State different types of partners. Explain any one.

b. Draw typical layout of retail drug store and mention its objectives.

c. Write factors affecting the selection of site for drug storage.

d. Define 'Retailer'. State the functions of pharmaceutical retailer.

e. Write procedure for disposal of scrap and surpuls.

Q 3. Answer any *three* of the following:

a. What is 'Joint Stock Company'? Give main features of it.

b. Write minimum requirements to start the drug store.

c. State various steps of purchase procedure.

d. Write factors affecting price determination.

e. Explain minimum and maximum stock levels.

Q 4. Answer any *three* of the following:

a. State the methods of evaluation of work performance of pharmacist.

b. Define 'Sales Promotion'. Explain the techniques of sales promotion.

c. Explain in brief EOQ.

d. State the advantages and disadvantages of market research.

e. Write factors affecting the selection of supplier.

Q 5. Answer any *three* of the following:

a. What is ABC analysis? State its advantages.

b. Define 'Budget'. State essentials of budgetary control.

c. Write important sources of the finance.

d. State the methods of compensation to the pharmacist.

e. State the methods of analysis of financial statement.

Q 6. Answer any *three* of the following:

a. State the objectives of book-keeping.

b. What is accounting concept? Explain separate entity and accrual conecpt of accountancy.

c. Give definition of trial balance and state the procedure for rectification of errors in trail balance.

d. Draw format of Profit and Loss Account and Balance Steet.

e. What is difference between journal and cash book?

Winter Examination 2010
D Pharm Second Year
Drug Store and Business Management

Q 1. Answer any *five* of the following:

   a. i. Define pharmaceutical management

      ii. Mention the various objectives of business.

   b. What is Govt. company, national and multinational company?

   c. What do you understand by "Hire Purchase Trading System"?

   d. Define Global and limited tender.

   e. Explain the graphic presentation of EOQ techniques of inventory control.

   f. What is shadow box display and high traffic display?

   g. What is bill of exchange and promissory note?

Q 2. Answer any *four* of the following:

   a. Give detailed classification of commerce.

   b. Mention the different kinds of partnership and partners. Explain them in brief.

   c. Mention any seven points of different between departmental store and multiple shops.

   d. What is mail order business? How is it utilized for pharmaceutical products?

   e. Mention any seven points of difference between private limited company and public limited company.

   f. What are the inflated, standard and replacement methods of pricing of materials for the purpose of dispensing?

Q 3. Answer any *four* of the following:

   a. What is codification? Explain the mnemonic and scientific methods of codification.

   b. Explain inventory carrying cost technique.

   c. What do you mean by legitimate scrap and defective scrap? Explain in brief scrap control and disposal of scrap.

   d. Give the expenses covered under procurement cost and carrying cost.

   e. How pharmaceutical sales promotion differs from the other product sales promotion? Explain the promition of

      i. Schedule products

      ii. Promotion of home remedies.

   f. Explain the postal and panel methods of survey in connection to market research.

Q 4. Answer any *four* of the following:

a. Write note on
   i. Job training   ii. Apprenticeship training

b. Give comparative data of current, fixed deposit and saving bank accountsl

c. Give comparative evolution of equity shares, preference shares and debentures.

d. Define letter of credit, overdue bills and negotiable instruments.

e. Classify organization of public enterprises and explain in brief departmental undertakings.

f. Explain itinerant retailers.

Q 5. Answer any *four* of the following:

a. Write note on analytical petty cash book.

b. What is purchase journal, sales journal, purchase return journal and sales return journal?

c. Explain:
   i. Total and balance method
   ii. Elimination of equal methods of trial balance.

d. Explain going concern concept and variable objective evidence concept.

e. What is compound journal entry and opening journal entry?

f. Mention five points of difference between profit and loss account and balance sheeet.

Q 6. Answer any *two* of the following:

a. Journalise the following transactions and post them into ledger.

1994	Particulars	Rs.
July 1	Ram commenced business with cash	12,000
July 2	Deposited into bank	9,000
July 3	Purchased good for cash	500
July 4	Bought furniture for office use	1,400
July 10	Drew from bank for office use	900
July 12	Goods sold to Kiran	700
July 16	Bought goods of Rahim	410
July 18	Paid trade expenses	100
July 19	Received cash from Kiran	590
	Allowed him Discount	10
July 24	Paid wages	40
July 28	Paid Rahim in full settlement	400
July 30	Paid rent	100
July 31	Interest on capital	100

b. Record the following transaction in Analytical Petty Cash Book.

1996	Particulars	Rs.
July 1	Amount received from head cashier	50.00
July 2	Purchased stationery	5.00
July 5	Postage	10.50
July 7	Printing charges	5.00
July 10	Paid tonga charges	1.00
July 14	Sent a telegram to thin and small	1.20
July 24	Printing charges	8.50
July 26	Purchased (Twine), Sutle, sua etc.	1.00
July 27	Paid cartage	0.50
July 30	Stationery purchased	1.25
July 30	For Rickshaw charges	0.50

c. Enter the following transactions in the three columnar cash book of M/s. Sanjay Medical Hall and balance it.

2008	Particulars	Rs.
April 1	Cash in hindi	10,000.00
	Cash in bank account	5,000.00
April 2	Received cash from Kunal	4,000.00
	Discount given	120.00
April 3	Paid into bank	3,000.00
April 4	Paid to Mauli and Co. by cheque	1,400.00
April 5	Received from cash sale	
	Cash	2,100.00
	Cheque	1,600.00
April 7	Paid for cash purchases by cheque	1,600.00
April 9	Paid by cheque to Maya and Sons in full settlement of Rs. 1,500.00	1,425.00
April 11	Drew for office use Personal use	1,000.00
April 14	Paid cash for advertisement	600.00
April 18	Drew a cheque for personal use	5,000.00
April 21	Paid life insurance premium	1,400.00
April 22	Paid rent	700.00
April 27	Paid salaries to staff by cheque	6,200.00
April 29	Received a cheque from M/s. Neid and Co. in full settlement of their A/c. for Rs. 6,200.00	5,800.00

d. From the information given below, prepare a Profit and Loss Account of M/s. Ravindra Medical Hall for the year ending March 31, 2007.

Particulars	Rs.
Gross profit	68,000.00
Rent	8,000.00
Salary	24,000.00
Commission paid	4,000.00
Interest on loan	3,000.00
Advertisement	7,000.00
Discount received	4,000.00
Printing and stationery	2,500.00
Legal charges	4,000.00
Bad debts	2,000.00
Depreciation	1,000.00
Interest received	8,000.00
Loss by fire	3,000.00

Summer Examination 2011
D Pharm Second Year
Drug Store and Business Management

Q 1. Solve any *five* of the following:

a. Define the terms (any *two*):
   i. Entrepot trade   ii. Profession
   iii. Small scale industry   iv. Firm
b. Explain the term 'Private company'.
c. Explain in brief 'Functional middlemen'.
d. Write two advantages and two disadvantages of opening a drug store in rural or small town.
e. Explain the meaning of Input–Output ratio.
f. State the various sources to collect long-term finance.

Q 2. Solve any *four* of the following:

a. Discuss various hindrances faced by a procedure in passing on its good to the consumers.
b. What functions do wholesalers perform?
c. Write the various documents needed to renew the license to sell drugs on wholesale.

d. Write the advantages of perpetual inventory system.

e. Discuss the various method used for advertising pharmaceutical products.

f. What is the purpose of giving training to newly recruited pharmacist?

Q 3. Solve any *four* of the following:

a. Give salient features of 'Joint Stock Company'.

b. What various methods would you suggest for an effective sales promotion campaign for the film which has shown decline in sales?

c. Differentiate between slow-moving, dormant materials and obsolete items.

d. Define the followint terms:

i.	Bin card	ii.	Recruitment
iii.	Finance	iv.	Fixed capital

e. Discuss the general factors to be considered while selecting a site for a drug store.

f. Write short note on Co-operative Banks.

Q 4. Solve any *four* of the following:

a. Differentiate between preference shares and ordinary shares.

b. What are the factors to be considered for the selection of supplier?

c. Explain various functions of management.

d. Differentiate between wholesaler and retailer.

e. Explain different methods of keeping the drugs in a retail store.

f. Define the following:

i.	Codification	ii.	Lead time
iii.	Business		

Q 5. Solve any *four* of the following:

a. Write disadvantages of mail order business.

b. What are the objectives of sales promotion?

c. Why is short term finance required? What are the main sources of raising it?

d. Define the following terms:

i.	Loan	ii.	Salesman
iii.	Trade		

e. What functions do C and F agents perform?

f. What are the different methods of pricing of materials for the purpose of dispensing?

Q 6. Solve any *four* of the following:

a. What do you understand by the term according? State objectives and branches of accounting.

   b. Differentiates between accounting concepts and accounting conventions with two examples of each.

   c. What do you understand by 'Books of Original Entry'? Explain main books of original entry in brief.

   d. What does the term 'Financial Statement' mean? Write its advantages and disadvantages.

   e. Explain 'Budgetary Control'. Mention requirement of effective 'Budgeting'.

   f. Explain the following terms:
      i. Activity ratio   ii. Liquidity ratio
     iii. Comparative financial analysis.

Winter Examination 2011
D Pharm Second Year
Drug Store and Business Management

Q 1. Attempt any *eight* of the following:

   a. Define the terms:
      i. Business   ii. Accounting

   b. Name the different types of accounts with examples and rules of 'debit and credit'.

   c. Write the advantages of Codification.

   d. Discuss the limitations of EOQ.

   e. Differentiate between overdraft and cash credit facility of commercial bank.

   f. Define cheque. State reasons for crossing cheque.

   g. State essential features of advertisement.

   h. Define trial balance. List the various errors which are not disclosed in Trial balance.

   i. Write the formula to calculate retail price of dug formulation.

   j. Define retailer. Name functions of retailer.

   K. Define and enlist techniques of sales promotion.

   l. State the minimum and maximum number of persons required to form:
      i. Private company   ii. Public company

Q 2. Answer any *four* of the following:

   a. Explain the qualities of good salesman.

   b. Define training. Discuss the various subjects to be covered during training to a pharmacist.

   c. Give the advantages and disadvantages of sole proprietorship business.

d. What is ABC techniques of inventory control?

e. Distinguish between departmental store and multiple shop

f. Define Budget. Discuss objectives of Budgetary control.

Q 3. Attempt any *four* of the following:

a. Define inventory. What are the main objectives of inventory control?

b. Define Trade. Write about Foreign Trade.

c. Mention the services rendered by wholesaler to producer and Retailer.

d. What is Joint Hindu Family Business? Explain its main features.

e. Define Merit Rating. How is evaluation of pharmacist done by 'Check List' method?

f. What are the objectives of purchasing?

Q 4. Attempt any four of the following:

a. Define book-keeping. Write advantages of double entry book-keeping system.

b. Enumerate accounting concepts. Explain 'Entity concept'.

c. Define Finance. Discuss various types of finance.

d. Explain various methods of preparation of trial balance.

e. Differentiate between Journal and Ledger.

f. Give the format of:
   i. Journal
   ii. Profit and loss account
   iii. Balance sheet

Q 5. Attempt any *four* of the following:

a. Define the terms:
   i. Posting
   ii. Asset
   iii. Liability

b. What is financial analysis? Discuss various methods of financial analysis.

c. Write about 'Petty Cash Book'.

d. Give examples of Subsidiary books. What are its necessities?

e. Discuss advantages and limitations of financial statements.

f. How will you include following items while preparing Profit and Loss account?
   i. Advertisement   ii. Loss of fire
   iii. Printing and stationery   iv. Interest
   v. Salary   vi. Rent

Q 6. Answer any *four* of the following:

a. Explain the various functions of management.

b. Write in detail about 'Scrap and Surplus' disposal.

c. Define the terms:
   i. Lead time ii. Economics
   iii. Tender iv. Debenture

d. Classify industry on the basis of types of the goods produced.

e. Define 'Market Research'. Enlist methods of market Research. Give its advantages.

f. Mention the various documents to be submitted for getting retail drug store licence. Draw an ideal layout design of retail drug store.

Summer Examination 2012
D Pharm Second Year
Drug Store and Business Management

Q 1. Attempt any *five* of the following:

a. Define (any *two*)
   i. International market ii. Primary market
   iii. Capital market

b. Define (any *four*)
   i. Capital ii. Proprietor
   iii. Transaction iv. Asset
   v. Account

c. Draw rulings of Journal and Ledger.

d. Mention four essential requisites of Budgetory Control.

e. Give formulae for
   i. Current ratio ii. Quick ratio

f. Give four characteristic features of cooperative form of organization.

g. Write four merits of Government Company Form of Business Organization.

Q 2. Attempt any *four* of following:

a. Give examples of any six Indian Nationalized Banks. Mention types of deposits received by Commercial Bank from public.

b. Give type of financial needs of a business.

c. Define business. Give essential features of business.

d. Give advantages and disadvantages of sole proprietorship business.

e. Define scrap. Give its classification. How scrap is accounted for?

f. Analyze the transaction:
i. Paid ₹ 2000 toward interest
ii. Purchased machinery worth ₹ 1000/- for cash
iii. Sold old furniture for ₹ 600/- for cash
iv. Received ₹ 5000/- on A/c from Mr. Wadekar.
v. Paid salary ₹ 3000/-

Q 3. Attempt any *four* of following:

a. Identify items of Trading A/c., P and L, and Balance Sheet from following:
i. Cash in hand and at Bank   ii. Drawings
iii. Purchases   iv. Salary
v. Rent and Taxes   vi. Capital
vii. Sales

b. Define cheque, Name parties to a cheque, give requisites to a cheque. What precautions must be taken by a person before drawing a cheque?

c. Give financial planning importance in case of a business enterprise.

d. Define trade, give its type; explain 'entrepot trade'.

e. Mention features of JHF firm. Give its advantages and disadvantages.

f. Mention different methods of inventory control. Give advantages of ABC method.

Q 4. Attempt any *four* of following:

a. From following data work out profitability ratios, i.e.
i. Gross profit ratio   ii. Operating ratio
iii. Operating profit ratio
iv. Net profit ratio in relation to sales;

Item	*(Figures in thousands)* Amount
Net sales	935
Cost of goods sold	582
Gross profit	353
Selling expenses	204
Administrative expenses	75
Total operating expenses	279
Operating profit	74
Other income	12
Other expenses	86
Income of the year before tax	11
Income tax	27
Net income for the year	48

    b. Mention factors to be considered for selecting a site for opening a new drug store.

    c. Mention types of middlemen; give four characteristics and four functions of wholesaler.

    d. Define sole proprietorship, mention its features.

    e. Define inventory control, write its objectives and functions.

    f. Define management, give its features, explain any two features.

Q 5. Attempt any *four* of the following:

    a. Mention financial service provided by following types of banks:
       i. Industrial bank
      ii. Savings bank
     iii. Exchange bank
     iv. Commercial bank

    b. Give sources of raising finance in case of following needs:
       i. Fixed capital
      ii. Working capital
     iii. Long term finance
     iv. Medium term finance
      v. Short term finance

    c. Mention principles of management.

    d. Define channel of distribution. How choice of channel of distribution is made?

    e. Differentiate between a wholesaler and retailer.

    f. Write about accounting principles.

Q 6. Attempt any *four* of following:

    a. Give main principles of double entry book-keeping system and rules of 'debit' and 'credit'.

    b. Define tender, mention different methods of obtaining tenders.

    c. Define purchasing; give its objective. Mention 4 'C's of credit information.

    d. Give different ownership forms of business organizations, mention factors of selecting a type of BO.

    e. Define market. Give classification of market.

    f. Explain following terms (any *three*):
       i. Trade credit
      ii. Cash credit
     iii. Bank overdraft
     iv. Public deposits
      v. Installment credit
     vi. Retained profit.

Winter Examination 2012
D Pharm Second Year
Drug Store and Business Management

Q 1. Solve any *eight* of the following:

   a. Define the terms:
        i. Industry   ii. Commerce
   b. Define the terms:
        i. Management   ii. Trade
   c. Mention different channels of distribution of drugs with intermediates.
   d. Give the diagram of Ideal layout for Retail Drug Store.
   e. Define the term condification of drugs. Name the different methods of codification.
   f. Define the term inventory control and enlist various inventory control techniques.
   g. What is EOQ? Give formula to calculate EOQ.
   h. Define the terms:
        i. Salesmanship   ii. Advertisement
   i. Explain the advantages of window display.
   j. Define the terms:
        i. Requirement   ii. Training
   k. Define the terms:
        i. Assest   ii. Liabilities
   l. Define the term cheque and mention different types of cheque.

Q 2. Solve any four:

   a. Define aids to trade. Discuss different aids to trade.
   b. What are the different forms of Business Organisation? Describe main features of sole proprietorship.
   c. Mention advantages and disadvantages of channels of distribution.
   d. Enlist the documents required to open a new medical retail drug store.
   e. Describe the ABC techniques of inventory control.
   f. What are the different qualities necessary to become a successful salesman?

Q 3. Solve any *four*:

   a. What are the various points and methods which should be taken into consideration for evaluation of pharmacist?
   b. Define bank. What are different kinds of bank? Mention secondary functions of bank.

   c. What do you understand by financial planning? What are the different sources of finance? Enlit them.

   d. Write a complete note on wholesaler of Drugs.

   e. How will you select site for opening new retail drug store?

   f. Mention the salient features of Hire purchase trading with its advantages and disadvantages.

Q 4. Solve any four:

   a. What are the different types of bank accounts? Mention various functions of bank.

   b. What do you understand by cooperative society? Mention various functions of bank.

   c. What do you mean by purchasing? Give its importance in growth of business.

   d. What do you mean by scrap? Describe the procedure for disposal of scrap and surplus.

   e. Define profit and loss A/c and give specimen format of profit and loss account.

   f. Mention the features and functions of management.

Q 5. Solve any *four*:

   a. Define balance sheet. Give specimen format of balance sheet.

   b. Name the various methods of financial analysis. Write a note on ratio analysis.

   c. Define the term Budget. What are the objectives of budgetary control?

   d. Explain the term ledger and its importance. Give specimen format of ledger.

   e. What do you understand by multiple shop system? Mention its advantages and disadvantages.

   f. Mention merits and various functions of retail trade of drugs.

Q 6. Solve any *four*:

   a. Define cash book. Mention different types of cash books with specimen format of all types of cash books.

   b. Define partnership. Mention different kinds of partners. Give advantages and disadvantages of partnership.

   c. Write a note on departmental stores. Mention its merits and demerits.

   d. Define the term tender and contract. Write a note on different types of tenders.

   e. Mention different methods of perpetual inventory control system. Give advantages and disadvantages of the system.

   f. What are the different account books? Enlist them. Mention advantages of Journal with its specimen format.

Summer Examination 2013
D Pharm Second Year
Drug Store and Business Management

Q 1. Answer any *eight* of the following:

   a. Define Commerce. Enlist various activities of Commerce.

   b. Define the term 'Business Organisation'. Write minimum four merits of sole proprietorship.

   c. Explain various channels of distribution of drugs.

   d. Explain the term contract. State various particulars to be mentioned in contract.

   e. Define inventory and state objectives of inventory control.

   f. Explain the term advertising. Enlist various media used for advertising pharmaceutical products.

   g. State and explain various types of Bank Accounts.

   h. State what you understand by books of origin entry. State various books of original entry.

   i. Write minimum four advantages of Hire Purchase Trading House.

   j. Define the term cheque. List out the salient features of cheque.

   k. State advantages of Perpetual Inventory Control System.

   l. Write objectives of sales promotion.

Q 2. Answer any *four* of the following:

   a. Define Accounting. State main objectives of Accounting.

   b. Write salient features of Joint Stock Company by giving six points.

   c. Explain in brief internal and international Trade.

   d. Differentiate between retailer and wholesaler with respect to their features, by giving six points.

   e. Explain the term Finance. State objectives of Financial management.

   f. Explain following terms:

      i. Training   ii. Recruitment

      iii. Partnership deed

Q 3. Answer any *four* of the following:

   a. Enlist various inventory control techniques. State advantages of ABC analysis.

   b. Explain the term sales promotion. Explain in brief any two sales promotion techniques.

   c. Explain the term industry. State classification of industries based on type of goods produced by them.

   d. Draw an ideal layout design of retail drug store and state objectives of layout design.

e. Differentiate between departmental stores and multiple shops.
f. Define scrap and surplus. State how scrap can be controlled in pharmaceutical industry.

Q 4. Attempt any *four* of the following:

a. State the formula to calculate retail price of a drug formulation. Explain FIFO and LIFO.
b. Explain the term codification of drugs. Explain methods of codification.
c. Define Salesmanship. State qualities a person should possess to become a successful salesman.
d. Explain 'Window Display' as one of the forms of advertisement.
e. Explain various kinds of partners in partnership form of business organisation.
f. Explain the following:
    i. Bank overdraft facility   ii. Cash credit facility
   iii. Industrial banks.

Q 5. Attempt any *four* of the following:

a. Explain different sources of finance.
b. Explain various points which has to be taken into consideration for evaluation of pharmacist.
c. Explain in brief VED analysis.
d. Define Tenders. Explain different types of Tenders.
e. Explain the steps necessary for purchasing.
f. Explain various functions of management.

Q 6. Attempt any *four* of the following:

a. State the format of Journal and Ledger, differentiate between Journal and Ledger.
b. Enlist types of cash book. Explain petty cash book alongwith its format.
c. Define trial balance. State objectives of trial balance and mention methods of preparing trial balance.
d. Explain the term Budget. Give classification of Budget. Explain Master Budget.
e. Enlist various forms of business organizations. State salient features of joint Hindu Family business by giving six points.
f. Explain the following terms:
    i. Transaction
   ii. Nominal account
  iii. Capital
  iv. Liquidity ratios

Winter Examination 2013
D Pharm Second Year
Drug Store and Business Management

Q 1. Solve any *eight* of the following:

a. State any four utility functions of the bank.

b. List our minimum requirements to start the retail drug store.

c. Define trade and classify trade.

d. State the main functions of pharmaceutical retailers.

e. Define industry. Classify industries with example of each class.

f. Write essential requirements of valid contract.

g. Give the objectives of inventory control.

h. Define partnership business. List the type of partners.

i. State the formula for calculating the retail price of drug formulations.

j. Define cheque and state different types of cheque.

k. List out the types of accounts with examples.

l. Define the following terms:
   i. Tender
   ii. Lead time

Q 2. Solve any *four* of the following:

a. Differentiate between a departmental stores and a multiple shops.

b. Draw ideal layout design for retail drug store. State objectives of layout design.

c. State the content of training programme designed for drug store pharmacist.

d. 'Advertisement is a social waste.' Give your comments.

e. Write the advantages of Budgetary control.

f. Write the financial sources available for fixed and working capital.

Q 3. Solve any *four* of the following:

a. State and explain the functions of management.

b. Explain the procedure followed for disposal of scrap and surplus items.

c. Write the methods of compensation of the pharmacist.

d. State the factors affecting the selection of supplier.

e. State advantages and disadvantages of advertisement of product.

f. State why window display is called silent salesman.

Q 4. Solve any *four* of the following:

a. What do you know about EOQ? State its methods.

b. State the salient features of Co-operative business.

   c. Explain money measurement and dual aspect concepts of accountancy.

   d. What is ABC techniques? Write its importance.

   e. State and explain aids used for removal of hindrances from Trade.

   f. Distinguish between Privateth Limited Company and Public Limited Company.

Q 5. Solve any *four* of the following:

   a. Explain C and F agent and state their importance in drug distribution.

   b. Define the terms:
      i. Capital
      ii. Bad debts
      iii. Safety stock

   c. Explain the qualities of good salesman.

   d. State commonly used means in analysing financial statements.

   e. State the different methods of preparation of Trail Balance.

   f. State salient features of Joint hindu family business.

Q 6. Solve any *four* of the following:

   a. What do you mean by cash book? Classify it. Write importance of petty cash book.

   b. Draw typical format of profit and loss account and balance sheet.

   c. State the difference between ledger and journal and draw a format for ledger and journal.

   d. State objectives of double entry system of book-keeping along with two advantages and disadvantages.

   e. Explain essential requisite of good financial planning.

   f. Journalize the following transactions:

Years 2010

1 April	–	Commenced business with cash ₹ 10,000/-
3 April	–	Bought goods for Rakesh on cash ₹ 2.750/-
5 April	–	Sold goods to Prakash on credit ₹ 1,650/-
10 April	–	Paid salaries of office staff of the month ₹ 830/-

Winter Examination 2014
D Pharm Second Year
Drug Store and Business Management

Q 1. Attempt any *eight* of the following:

   a. What is supply order?

   b. What is bill of exchange and promissory note?

   c. Define:
      i. Business
      ii. Management
   d. Explain Hire-Purchase trading system.
   e. Mention different channels of distribution of drugs with intermediates.
   f. Write the formula to calculate retail price of drug formulation.
   g. Draw ideal layout design for retail drug store.
   h. What is Entreport trade?
   i. What is Master Budget?
   j. Define:
      i. Liabilities
      ii. Assets
   k. What is mail order business?
   l. Define banking and enlist types of banks.

Q 2. Attempt any *four* of the following:

   a. Define:
      i. Safety stock level
      ii. Reorder level
      iii. Maximum stock level
   b. Define wholesaler. Explain functions of wholesaler.
   c. How will you select site for opening new drug store?
   d. Define aids to trade and explain activities revolving around trade.
   e. Differentiate between preference shares and ordinary shares.
   f. Define recruitment and explain methods of recruitment.

Q 3. Attempt any *four* of the following:

   a. Define:
      i. Slow moving materials.
      ii. Dormant materials.
      iii. Obsolete items.
   b. Explain postal and panel methods of survey in connection to market research.
   c. Define and explain types of scrap.
   d. Differentiate between private company and public company.
   e. Explain itinerant retailers.
   f. Give the documents required to open a wholesale drug store.

Q 4. Attempt any *four* of the following:

   a. Discuss ABC analysis of inventory control.
   b. Enlist and explain functions of management.
   c. Explain codification methods of items in drug store.

    d. Discuss salient features of Joint Hindu Family Business.

    e. Write the selection procedure to select pharmacist.

    f. Explain the qualities of good salesman.

Q 5. Attempt any *four* of the following:

    a. Enlist the advantages and disadvantages of co-operative society.

    b. Discuss the services of commercial banks.

    c. Define and classify Budget.

    e. Define trial balance and explain rectification of errors.

    f. Explain the compensation methods to pharmacist.

Q 6. Attempt any *four* of the following:

    a. Differentiate between profit and loss account and balance sheet.

    b. Discuss the following:

        i. Accrual concept

        ii. Money measurement concept.

    c. Journalise the following transactions.

April 2012	₹
1 Started Business with cash	10,000
2 Bought medicines for cash	5,000
3 Sold medicines to Ram	3,000
5 Sold medicines for cash	4,000
6 Received cash from Ram	2,500
13 Purchased furniture from Deva	2,400
18 Paid for shop rent	500
20 Purchase medicine from Kumar	3,500
30 Cash paid to Girish	1,000
30 Receive commission	500

    d. What do you mean by Cash Book? Classify it.

    e. Explain the terms:

        i. Overdraft facility.

        ii. Cash credit facility.

    f. Discuss the profitability ratios.

Summer Examination 2015
D Pharm Second Year
Drug Store and Business Management

Q 1. Attempt any *eight* of the following:

    a. Define:
        i. Industry
        ii. Management

    b. State various middlemen in trade.

    c. Draw a typical layout design of retail drug store.

    d. State advantages and disadvantages of opening a drug store in rural area or small town.

    e. Enlist various inventory control techniques.

    f. Define term sales promotion and state any four objectives of sales promotion.

    g. Define bank and enlist various kinds of banks.

    h. State any four advantages of budgetary control.

    i. Define accounting and state any two objectives of accounting.

    j. Enlist various accounting concepts.

    k. State any four advantages of perpetual inventory system.

    l. State various aspects to be covered during training of a pharmacist.

Q 2. Attempt any *four* of the following:

    a. Give classification of budget.

    b. What are various sources of finance?

    c. Explain various types of trade.

    d. State and explain various types of partners in partnership form of business.

    e. Differentiate between a departmental stores and a multiple shop.

    f. Define the term advertising. Discuss various media for advertising.

Q 3. Attempt any *four* of the following:

    a. Explain various methods of codification of drugs in a drug store.

    b. What do you mean by EOQ? Enlist various methods of EOQ. Explain any one method.

    c. Discuss various methods of compensating a pharmacist so as to retain him on the job.

    d. What are the limitations of economics?

    e. Mention salient features of co-operative society.

    f. Explain importance of window display for retail drug store.

Q 4. Attempt any *four* of the following:

a. Explain the terms:
   i. Debentures   ii. Ploughing back of profit
   iii. Cheque
b. State advantages and disadvantages of mail order business.
c. Define tenders. Explain various types of tenders.
d. Explain ABC techniques of inventory control.
e. Explain various methods of market research.
f. Discuss the role played by banking, transport and insurance to facilitate trade.

Q 5. Attempt any *four* of the following:

a. Differentiate between joint stock company and partnership firm.
b. Define the term purchase procedure and explain various steps in purchase procedure.
c. Define retailers and state various functions of retailers.
d. Give functions of bank.
e. Explain the terms:
   i. Transaction   ii. Nominal account
   iii. Assets
f. Define scrap and give its classification.

Q 6. Attempt any *four* of the following:

a. Define cash book. State types of cash book. Explain petty cash book along with its format.
b. Define balance sheet. Draw its format and state how it differs from profit and loss account.
c. Define trial balance and discuss methods of preparing trial balance.
d. Give the format of journal and ledger. Differentiate between journal and ledger.
e. Name various methods of financial analysis. Write in short about analysis.
f. Journalise the following transaction for ABC medical store:

Year 2014	Particulars	Amount ₹
1stJan	Purchased goods for cash	50,000
3rd Jan	Purchased furniture	25,000
5th Jan	Sold goods for cash	5,000
7th Jan	Received from D'souza	2,000
7th Jan	Sold goods to Mukesh	5,000
9th Jan.	Paid rent	2,500
20th Jan	Paid salaries	10,000
25th Jan	Deposited into bank	7,000

Winter Examination 2015
D Pharm Second Year
Drug Store and Business Management

Q 1. Solve any *eight* of the following:

a. State the limitations of budgetary control.

b. What is cash book? List out various types of cash book.

c. State how inventory carrying cost of business can be reduced.

d. Define the term:
   i. Contract
   ii. Safety stock

e. What is retailer? State different types of pharmaceutical retailers.

f. Enlist the documents enclosed with Form 19 for obtaining the drug licence.

g. Define tender. Write the types of tender used in the market.

h. State the difference between overdraft and cash credit facility offered by the bank.

i. State types of accounts with suitable examples.

j. State why profit and loss account is prepared.

k. Classify different types of business organisations with example of each class.

l. Write the difference between departmental store and multiple shop.

Q 2. Solve any *four* of the following:

a. What is ABC technique of analyzing the inventory? Write its advantages.

b. Give common methods of drug codification. State their advantages and disadvantages.

c. State the different aids to trade.

d. Distinguish between private and public limited company.

e. Write the sources of finance required to fulfil working capital of business.

f. State how will you select the site for retail drug store.

Q 3. Solve any *four* of the following:

a. Write the functions of management.

b. Draw an ideal layout design for retail drug store.

c. State various medias of advertising the product in market.

d. Write the qualities of good salesman.

e. Define industry. State various types of manufacturing industry.

f. State the main features of co-operative business.

Q 4. Solve any *four* of the following:

a. State various methods òf economic order quantity calculation..

b. 'Window display acts as silent salesman'. Give your comments.

c. Write the content of training programme designed for drug store pharmacist.

d. State the functions of C & F agent.

e. Write the objectives of double entry system of book keeping.

f. Define recruitment. State the factors affecting the process of Recruitment.

Q 5. Solve any *four* of the following:

a. Write the procedure followed for disposal of scrap and surplus in market.

b. State the methods compensation to pharmacist.

c. Define bank. State the types of accounts the bank provides to its customers.

d. What do you understand by 'market research'? State its objectives.

e. What is financial statement? State the methods of analyzing the financial statement.

f. Define balance sheet. State the character and purpose of preparation of balance sheet.

Q 6. Solve any *four* of the following:

a. Write public utility functions of the bank.

b. State various steps involved in purchasing.

c. What do you know about the book of original entry? Draw its specimen format.

d. Write the steps involved in rectification of errors present in trial balance.

e. Journalise the following transactions:

1st April, 2005	– Ram started business with cash ₹ 5,000.
3rd April, 2005	– Bought goods from Sharma ₹ 750.
8th April, 2005	– Sold goods to Rakesh on cash ₹ 1,375 discount allowed ₹ 25.
9th April, 2005	– Paid rent to landlord ₹ 300

f. Prepare simple cash book from the following:

1st Jan, 2010	– Commenced business with cash ₹ 15,000.
7th Jan, 2010	– Purchased goods from Satyanarayan on cash ₹ 2,350.
11th Jan,2010	– Sold goods to Saket ₹ 950.
19th Jan, 2010	– Received cash from Saket ₹ 500.
26th Jan, 2010	– Bought goods from Patel & Co. on credit ₹ 1,600.
31st Jan, 2010	– Paid salary of the month ₹ 1,200.

Summer Examination 2016
D Pharm Second Year
Drug Store and Business Management

Q 1. Solve any *eight* of the following:

a. Define the term:
  i. Commerce
  ii. Consumer goods
b. Define the term 'cheque'. Give three parties to a cheque.
c. Write the importance of warehouse by giving minimum four points.
d. What is mean by 'books of original entries'? Give two examples of it.
e. Explain functional middleman with two examples.
f. Define 'evaluation'. What is the need of evaluation of employees?
g. What is meaning of accounting concepts and convention in accountancy?
h. Write the difference between journal and ledger.
i. What is a meaning of contra entry'? Why contra entry is not posted in ledger? Give reason.
j. What is 'ordering cost' and 'inventory carrying cost'?
k. Define' purchasing'. Write objectives of purchasing.
1. Enlist minimum four techniques of inventory control.

Q 2. Solve any *four* of the following:

a. Give classification of trade. Write any four advantages of internal trade.
b. Define 'share'. Explain different types of share.
c. Give the format of balance sheet. Explain methods of marshalling of balanc sheet.
d. Enlist various kinds of partners. Explain 'minor partner' in detail.
e. What is petty cash book? Explain working of petty cashier.
f. What is pharmaceutical management? Enlist different levels of management. Give any two functions performed by middle level management.

Q 3. Solve any *four* of the following:

a. What is 'partnership deed'? Give any four features of partnership organisation.
b. Enlist various sites to open retail drug store. According to you which sites are good sites to open new retail drug store? Give reason.
c. Explain the term 'budgetary control'. Discuss various objectives of budgetary control.

    d. What does the term 'financial statement' mean? Write two advantages and two disadvantages of it.

    e. Define the term (any *three*):
      i. Bad debts
      ii. Lead time
      iii. Buffer stock
      iv. Capital

    f. Enlist various methods used for advertising pharmaceutical products. Explain outdoor advertisement of general and home remedies product.

Q 4. Solve any *four* of the following:

    a. Differentiate between current A/c, savings A/c and fixed deposit A/c on the basis of the following points:
      i. Withdrawals
      ii. Restriction on operation
      iii. Interest

    b. Explain salient features of sole trading business organisation by giving minimum six points.

    c. Define aids to trade. List its auxiliaries. Explain importance of transportation in commerce.

    d. Define 'tender'. Explain various kinds of tender.

    e. Define the term 'trial balance'. Explain various errors in account, which are present but not reflected in trial balance.

    f. Define 'market research'. Explain various methods of market research.

Q 5. Solve any *four* of the following:

    a. Explain 'departmental store'. Write its two advantages and two disadvantages.

    b. Give any six salient features of retailer.

    c. Draw an ideal layout design for retail drug store. Write any four objectives of layout design.

    d. Explain going concern concept and money measurement concept of accountancy.

    e. Define 'industry'. Give classification of industry. Explain heavy industry and light industry.

    f. Explain various qualities of a good salesman.

Q 6. Solve any *four* of the following:

    a. Define codification. Explain different methods used for codification.

    b. Define ledger. Give the format of it. Explain the process of balancing of ledger account.

c. Explain in detail about different types of accounts in accountancy with their golden rules.

d. Define 'inventory Control'. Explain ABC technique of inventory control.

e. Define Selection. What steps are involved in selection of employee?

f. Journalise the following transactions of M/s Milind Medical Hall for the month of Jan 2014:

Jan 1	Started business with cash ₹ 1,00,000
Jan 4	Bought goods worth ₹ 40,000
Jan 7	Sold goods worth ₹ 20,000
Jan 10	Sold goods to Patel ₹ 15,000
Jan 19	Goods worth ₹ 5,000 returned from Patel
Jan 31	Received ₹ 10,000 from Patel

Winter Examination 2016
D Pharm Second Year
Drug Store and Business Management

Q 1. Solve any *four* of the following:

a. Define partners by holding out.

b. What is government company?

c. What is del credere agent?

d. Define open tender and global tender.

e. What is lead time?

f. What is sky writing?

g. What is land development bank?

Q 2. Solve any *four* of the following:

a. Mention different kinds of partnership and explain partner by estoppel.

b. Mention different kinds of company and explain company limited by guarantee.

c. Differentiate between company and partnership firm.

d. Differentiate between firm multiple shop and departmental stores.

e. What do you understand by hire purchase trading system? Mention its advantage and disadvantage.

f. What is joint hindu family business? Write its salient features.

Q 3. Solve any *four* of the following:

a. What are the legal requirements to run the drug store?

b. Explain different methods of pricing of materials.

   c. What is scrap? Mention different types of scrap and explain scrap control and disposal of scrap.

   d. Define codification. What are the methods of codification?

   e. What do you understand by V.E.D. analysis?

   f. What are the various functions of management?

Q 4. Solve any *four* of the following:

   a. What is advertising and what are different methods of advertising?

   b. Explain different techniques of sales promotion.

   c. Give different sources of recruitment.

   d. What is selection and write the selection procedure for appointment of pharmacist

   e. Explain the various services of commercial banks.

Q 5. Solve any *four* of the following:

   a. What is bank reconciliation statement and negotiable instruments?

   b. What is trade? Give classification of trade.

   c. Define mortgages, debenture, equity shares.

   d. What is assets? Explain different types of assets.

   e. What is imprest system? Write note on analytical petty cash book.

   f. What is difference between journal and ledger?

Q 6. Solve any *four* of the following:

   a. What are different methods used for financial analysis?

   b. Explain three columnar cash book.

   c. Write the different arithmetical errors in trial balance.

   d. What is going concern concept, realization concept?

   e. Write the rules of journalising.

   f. Define budgetary control. Give classification of budgets.

Summer Examination 2017
D Pharm Second Year
Drug Store and Business Management

Q 1. Solve any *eight* of the following:

   a. Define the terms:
      i. Commerce
      ii Business

   b. Enlist various forms of business organizations.

   c. Define accounting. Give two objectives of accounting.

   d. Explain different account types in accounting with examples.

   e. Enlist various types of partners in partnership firm of business.

f. Give any four salient features of co-operative society form of business.

g. State channels of distribution for pharmacy.

h. Explain the objectives of inventory control in short.

i. State what do you mean by cash book and enlist various types of cash book.

j. Define bank and enlist various kinds of banks.

k. State objectives of sales promotion.

l. Define the terms:

    i. Safety stock

    ii. Lead time

Q 2. Solve any *four* of the following:

a. Define scrap. Explain various types of scrap and how can the scrap be controlled.

b. Give detail classification of retailers. Explain itinerant retailers.

c. Define market research. Enlist methods of market research and give any two advantages of market research.

d. State the difference between joint stock company and partnership firm.

e. Explain various branches of accounting.

f. Mention the salient features of hire purchase trading with its advantages and disadvantages.

Q 3. Solve any *four* of the following:

a. Explain types of financial needs of business.

b. State and explain different methods of perpetual inventory control.

c. Define codification of drugs. State and explain various methods of drug codification.

d. State what do you mean by budgetory control. Give its advantages.

e. Explain what do you mean by slow-moving, dormant and obsolete items.

f. Differentiate between departmental stores and a multiple store.

Q 4. Solve any *four* of the following:

a. Explain various activities which revolves around trade.

b. Define sale proprietorship, mention its features.

c. Define advertisement. State any four advantages and disadvantages of advertisement of product.

d. Explain various points which have to be taken into consideration for valuation of pharmacist.

e. State and explain minimum, legal requirements for starting a retail drug store.

f. Explain the process of purchase followed in business organisation.

Q 5. Solve any *four* of the following:

a. Explain the functions of management.

b. Explain in detail ABC technique of inventory control.

c. Explain the following terms:
   i. Management
   ii. Economics
   iii. Recruitment

d. Explain any four techniques of sales promotion.

e. Enlist and explain how long-term finance be raised.

f. Explain the term budget. Give classification of budget.

Q 6. Solve any *four* of the following:

a. Explain the terms accounting concept and convention. Enlist various concepts and conventions.

b. Explain the term ledger, give its importance, draw format of ledger.

c. Differentiate between balance sheet and profit and loss A/c.

d. State how will you select the ideal site of drug store in urban as well as rural area.

e. Define financial analysis and explain profitability ratio.

f. Journalise the following transaction for the year 2016:

Jan 1	Neeraj invest ₹ 50,000 in cash.
Jan 5	Buys furniture for ₹ 20,000 on credit from Mr. Naresh.
Jan 15	Purchases goods for ₹ 10,000 from Mr. Naik.
Jan 16	Withdraws money ₹ 5,000 for personal use.
Jan 18	Receives cash ₹ 3,000 from Gopal.
J an 20	Issue cheques of ₹ 1,000 in favour of landlord for rent.
Jan 2	Sold goods for ₹ 6,000 to Mr. Nitin.
Jan 29	Pays salary to staff ₹ 10,000.